Bedtime Stories for Kids

Fun and Calming Tales for Your Children to Help Them Fall Asleep Fast! Helping Out and other beautiful stories!

Sleep Academy

Helping Out

"MOM!! DAD!!" I called at the top of my lungs. Flash and I had been sitting in the sandbox playing around when he kicked my sandcastle down. I had worked hard on that!

Dad came walking out with Mommy. Mom had her around Dad and was leaning against him as they walked.

"What's the matter, Anne?" Mom asked me. "Flash kicked down my sandcastle!" I complained and pointed at the ruins of my once happy kingdom. "Castle Anne was completely finished! Then Flash knocked it down! The kingdom of love and loyalty is now nothing!" I complained loudly.

Dad and Mom took a seat in the grass outside of the sandbox. "Where's Flash now?" Daddy asked me. "He ran away as soon as I called you," I growled and pointed down the road.

"Suppose you want me to go find him?" Dad asked me. "Duh!" I said to him. "You want me to ground him or yell at him?" I nodded as Daddy picked me up. He tickled my belly, and I began to scream out my laughter.

"DADDY!! St-St-Stop it!!" I giggled, but then Mom began to tickle me as well. "St-Stop! I can't breathe!"

They slowly let me go, and then Dad stood up and grabbed a large stick. "Here, Ames. I'll be right back." Mom grabbed the stick, and shakily pulled herself up.1

"Come here, Anne," Mommy said and picked me up. She held me on her hip, and I clung around her waist tightly. Dad ran down the driveway as Mom giggled at me. "You wanna hear a quick story while Dad's gone?" Mom asked me. I nodded, ecstatic, for what only I would hear.

"A year or two ago, your father was holding you and your brother. We went outside to show you two this sandbox, but on his way, he dropped your brother."

I blurted out, laughing hysterically. "Really? HA! No wonder Flash's a-"

I stopped myself before I could continue my sentence. "Let's go inside, okay?" My mom said, but she sounded weird. "Are you okay, Mommy?" I asked her. She nodded but winced as we walked inside. "Uncle Tails, Knuckles, and Aunt Zooey and Sticks are coming over today." She told me.

"Really! I haven't seen them in forever!" I screamed. "Your father and I will be going for a walk for a short while. Those four are going to take care of you."

"Flash is gonna be here too... Isn't he?" I asked. "Of course, he's your brother."

The doorbell rang, and I ran to answer it. It was Dad who was holding Flash in his arms. "Apologize to your sister, Flash." He said sternly.

"..." Flash remained silent and crossed his arms.

"Flash!" Dad yelled at him.

"Fine, I'm sorry..." He said, and Dad sat him down.

I accepted his apology and then told him about who was coming over.

Once our family got here, Mom and Dad left. But we didn't really see them leave.

Walking

Together

It had been a long day, and Sonic and I were finally putting Anne and Flash to bed. "How was your walk?" Flash asked us. "It was relaxing. Your father and I enjoy our time alone, but you two make us extremely happy." I answered and kissed Flash's nose. He wiggled his nose, which happened to look like his father's.

"What'd you two talk about? Did you walk okay, Mommy?" Anne asked us next. "We talked a lot about you two. How you two are so special and important to us." Sonic told them sweetly. That was only partially true.

We talked about them, but we mostly talked about how we'll protect them. "Okay, will you tell us a story?" Anne and Flash asked us together. I sighed, as did Sonic. "Sorry, you two. We're worn out. You think you can go without a story?" Anne looked at me and seemed to see how tired I was. Then she looked at Sonic, who seemed just as tired as I.

"Okay..." Anne sighed, sounding disappointed. Flash heaved a sigh; he sounded so dismal and upset. I bit my lip as Sonic was heading to the door.

"You know- I could stay and tell a quick story?" Sonic turned to me, and he was very superstitious about this idea. "Ames, I don't think it's a good idea. You need this rest." I crossed my arms and shook my head. "That's an exaggeration; I don't need to sleep yet. Our two precious babies need their story." I grinned at him. Sonic sighed and sat down on the floor at the door.

"I'm staying right here." He declared. I grinned and went over to him. I sat down in his lap, and he kissed my face.

"Okay, so this is just a quick story. While your father and I were walking around outside, we saw this moose. It looked cross-eyed. It reminded us of this time; Sticks went crazy about this curse thing. We had to go find this monkey to cure her. The monkey was a fake, and it made us do all its chores. It drove us all insane!"2

Sonic grinned at the quick story and then stood up. I stood up, with the help of Sonic, and we went off to our beds.

I HATE that faker

"Dad? Who's Shadow?" Flash asked me. "Shadow? Uh... an old friend. Why'd you ask?" I asked him. "Mom was talking about him a few times today." My senses grew alert, and my ears pulled back. "Was she now?" I said, sat by Anne's bed. "Yeah, she said she dated him once. Then when she started dating you, he came back, and you scared him."

"Why is Amy talking about Shadow?" I thought as the door opened. Amy walked in with water glasses, and I glared at her. "So Ames, anything you wanna say? Anything about Shadow?" I asked her. "Oh, that's right, he's coming over for dinner tomorrow. I almost forgot." She laughed. "How do you forget something like that?!" I thought angrily.

"Daddy! Can we hear another story about Mr. Shads?" Anne asked as Flash covered his ears. "I don't like Shadow. He dated our mom; Dad's the only one that's supposed to date Mom." Flash growled at Anne. "But Mr. Shads looks cute from the photo I saw in the attic!" Anne whined.

"Photo?"

"Let me see the photo, Anne," I said to her. She pulled out an old photo that had Shadow and I in it. Amy looked over my shoulder and smiled. "That was one of the days you two didn't fight." She smiled. "That was because you were with us that day," I told her and handed Anne the photo.

"Okay, a story about Ol' Shads. Let's see... Amy and I were probably just a few months into dating..."

• • • • •

Sonic kissed Amy on the cheek, and Amy giggled at him. "Oh, Sonic... You're just the sweetest." Amy grinned at him. They were on the beach together, and no one else was around.

Or so they thought...

"Sonic!" They heard an angry voice call from behind them. Sonic turned around and saw Shadow running towards them, preparing for an attack. Sonic grabbed Amy quickly and jumped away from his attack.

"What's your problem?!" Sonic hissed and stood in front of Amy to protect her. "I was supposed to get paid if I fought you last time. I wasn't able to because of your stupid Dark Form!" Shadow growled. "You ruined my chance to get my money!" Shadow hissed at him.

"He's upset over money?" Sonic thought but stayed on guard. "You were going to hurt Amy! My Ames! My Flower!" Sonic yelled in his defense, and his fur stood on edge.

"Flower? Very generic, Faker!" Shadow laughed. Sonic had had enough of Shadow now. "Why don't you just shut up and go back to where you came from?!" Sonic yelled and rushed towards Shadow, ready to punch him.

Shadow dodged and landed across from Sonic as Sonic slid back around to face Shadow. Shadow teleported above Sonic and was about to hit him on the head when Sonic flipped on his back and kicked Shadow across the beach. Sonic waited to see if Shadow would stand up and throw a blow. It was all quiet until Shadow began to stir in the sand. He stood up with hatred burning in his eyes. Sonic simply smirked, ready for any type of attack.

But instead of Shadow heading straight for Sonic, he made a turn at the last second. "What?" Sonic thought, then looked back. "Amy!" Sonic raced to catch up to Shadow.

"LEAVE HER ALONE!!" Sonic yelled, and he ran faster than he ever had, and he jumped and grabbed Shadow's quills. They both went tumbling to the sand as Sonic pulled on Shadow's quills.

"Hey!! Ow!! Stop that!! That hurts!!" Shadow whined and tried to slap Sonic. "You little pest!" Shadow hissed and grabbed Sonic's own quills.

"You two stop!" Sonic and Shadow both let go of each other's quills as Amy grabbed their ears. "Hey! What are you doing that to me? Shadow started it!" Sonic yelled out. "You two are acting like children! Shadow, you leave NOW, or I'll make Dark Sonic come out !" Sonic and Shadow both widened their eyes. "You can do that?" They asked. "Yes, now Shadow, LEAVE!!" Shadow bolted away as soon as Amy let him go.

Then Amy let Sonic and go, and he rubbed his ear to ease the pain. "Can you really make 'him' come out?" Sonic asked Amy. Amy nodded at him. "But I won't tell you how or do it unless it's necessary." She smiled at him. Sonic nodded and hung his head. "Sorry for going off on Shadow. He just- struck a nerve, you know?" Sonic chuckled embarrassingly. Amy kissed Sonic quickly on the lips. "It's okay; I'm not mad at you. Your ears are just too cute, and I wanted to pinch them!" Amy giggled.

•••••

"Eww, Daddy, that's weird!" Flash said and pretended to retch. "Shadow isn't very nice, is he?" Anne asked me. I shook my head. "He's changed, though." Amy quickly added. "He even has given money to charities." She smiled. I rolled my eyes. "Be prepared, kids. Alright, goodnight." I smiled at them, and Amy and I kissed their heads.

We turned off the light and cracked the door, then finally went to our room.

Mommy and Daddy time

I shut the door behind Sonic, and Sonic launched himself onto me. We had just put the kids to bed, and they were fast asleep. Sonic's lips were against mine, and we kissed for what seemed like forever.

"Oh, Sonic..." I said between breaths.

"Ames..." He said slowly. "We haven't done this in so long..." He said as he pushed me closer to his body.

"I love you, Sonic. But you know we can't... not now..." I told him. Sonic sighed and nodded after he gave me a one kiss on my neck.+

"The kids aren't ready for a little sister or brother yet. We have to think of them." I told him sweetly. Sonic nodded, but he looked aggravated. "He really was looking forward to this. This is our anniversary, after all." I thought and flipped to my side. I made outlines of circles in Sonic's chest fur that had grown out.1

"Why don't we go out for something? We'll call Tails and Zooey over to take care of those two." I suggested to Sonic in my sweetest and most romantic voice. "Where would we go? The theaters closed, the restaurants aren't going to be open by the time we get there." Sonic really was upset over this.

"SooOOooOoonic..." I said in a singsong voice. "Yes, Amy?" He said. "Stop being mad. I know this night isn't how you pictured it going, but this can still work out." I said and cuddled my face into his shoulder. "No, no, it's okay. Let's just sleep." Sonic said, but he sounded angry. I sat up and jumped out of bed. "Ames?" Sonic sat up and watched me as I stormed out of our room.

I sat by myself in the living room for a few minutes before Sonic came in and wrapped an arm around me. "Sweetie, I didn't mean it like that. I'm sorry, Ames." Sonic apologized and rubbed my back. "I know you didn't mean it that way. It's just that... I feel like you blame me for-"

"Blame you? Oh no, Ames, no, I could never blame you for anything." Sonic said and kissed my cheek. "How about- I feel like you don't understand where I'm coming from. We can't take care of three kids, not yet anyway. I don't want to take the chance, Sonic."

"It's okay, it's okay, Ames. I was just upset and was caught up in the moment. I understand now." I shuddered as Sonic stood up and picked me up. "Let's go back to our rooms now, okay?" I nodded, and he took me back to our room.

Scary Story

"You all ready for a scary story?" I smiled at Anne and Flash. The kids nodded excitedly.

"Ok, this is a true story, Daddy and Mommy, okay?" Sonic said to them. They nodded at him and smiled. "Ok, let's start."

•••••

Sonic stared at Amy as Eggman grabbed her wrist. "Don't you dare touch her!" Sonic shouted angrily. "I'll break her just like you break my robots!" Eggman smirked and squeezed Amy's wrist tightly. "Oww!! Let me go!!" Amy growled and kicked Eggman, but he wouldn't release her.

"Stop!!!" Sonic screamed and cried out. "Robots! Grab him!" Eggman ordered, and robots grabbed hold of Sonic's legs. "Let me go!! Amy, I'm coming!!" Sonic yelled.

"Don't worry, Sonic. I'll b-be fine!" Amy winced as Eggman squeezed tighter. It felt like her hand was breaking. Amy screamed in pain.

Sonic growled angrily as a dark aurora began to flow around him. "Don't... Amy..." Sonic's fur grew dark, and he was filled with rage. "This is why I was scared of dating her. She'd get hurt; I took a chance. I won't let this happen again!" Sonic screamed inside his head.

Sonic punched and kicked the robots away from him. "Give me my Amy!!" He screamed. Eggman yelped but didn't move. "GIVE ME AMY NOW!!!" Sonic shouted at the top of his lungs. Eggman's grip was released, and Amy fell to the ground carelessly.

Sonic flew down and grabbed Amy. Eggman escaped while Sonic strokes Amy lovingly. "Ames? You're okay, right?" Sonic's heart was beating with so much rage and sadness. "S-Sonic?" Amy opened her eyes and let out a small yelp. She hadn't expected Sonic to be like this when she woke up. "I'm sorry, I know I'm scared; I need help calming down. Eggman, he hurt you! I-I can't-" Sonic's voice was stuttered and scared.

"Sonic, look at me." Amy smiled at him. "I'm not seriously hurt. My hand might be broken, but I'm okay. Calm down." She smiled and rubbed her button nose against his. "Okay, Ames."

•••••

Anne and Flash both glared at me. "What?" I smiled at them. "That wasn't scary!" They complained. "You left out bits too!" Flash whines and crossed his arms. "Well, some parts weren't right for your age. You'll hear the whole story when you're older." I told them. They huffed, and I kissed their heads. "Goodnight, sweeties." I smiled warmly at them. "Night, dad!"

That Awkward
Moment

"Mommy, can you tell us about the dinner you, Daddy, and Mr. Shads had?" Anne asked me. I tilted my head in confusion. "You were there, Anne," I told her. "Yeah... But not for all of it. What did you all talk about?" She asked me. Flash lifted an eyebrow, obviously interested too.

"Well, alright, I suppose I could tell you about our conversation." I shrugged at them. "I warn you; it wasn't anything spectacular..."

•••••

"So you and Rose have two little ones, now?" Shadow asked as he peeked into the living room where Anne and Flash were watching TV happily together.

"Yeah, Anne and Flash, their twins if you hadn't realized," Sonic answered him, but in a rude tone. Shadow glares his eyes, ready to start a fight if necessary.

"So, Shadow, how has your life been?" I stepped between them and smiled warmly. Shadow shrugged his shoulders. "Eh, it's as good a life an immortal can live." He said, still expressionless.

Sonic, who obviously forgot Shadow was never one to show emotion, thought he was rude.

"You could be a little nicer to my wife, Shadow," Sonic said protectively, but Amy glared at Sonic to be quiet. "Shadow is a very nice guest, Sonic. Why don't we start dessert?" Amy smiled and blushed, desperate to change the subject.

"DESSERT?!" Flash and Anne screamed from the living room. Shadow eyed Flash and Anne as they ran in, quick as lightning, and begged for ice cream.

Sonic kept a close eye on Shadow. He was looking for him to mess up so he could throw him out. Anne and Flash ate their dessert, and then Anne walked over to Shadow.

"Hey, Mr. Shads. I was wondering if you'd like to play connect 4 with us?" She asked him. Shadow raised an eyebrow at her. He hadn't expected her to ask him of all people to play a game. "Very well, how do you play?" He asked her. Anne grinned and grabbed Shadow's wrist. She pulled him into their living room happily.

•••••

"And that's all that happened." Amy smiled at them. "That...wasnot as interesting as I thought it would be..." Anne and Flash said, disappointment filling their voices. "Well, I did warn you two," Amy told them and kissed their foreheads. "Night, sweeties." Amy grinned and left a crack in the door. "Love you, mommy! Night!"

Cute Annoyance

I flopped down in Amy and I's bed. "Those two take forever to get to bed," I stated and flipped to my side so I could look at Amy. Amy flipped away from me as I did. "What?" I immediately grew concerned. "What did I do? I thought I was the perfect husband and dad today!" I thought and sat back up.

"Ames?" I asked and rubbed her shoulder. "You okay?" I asked her. Amy shrugged her shoulder away from me. "What did I do this time?" I thought to myself. Amy sat up and crossed her arms. She sat on the edge of the bed and stuck her nose in the air. She obviously wasn't in the mood for talking.

"Who cares if she's in the mood or not? I'm her husband! I should be able to talk to her whenever I want!" I growled lowly to myself.

"Ames? What did I do? Are you mad at me? Talk to me, Ames..." I had both my hands on her shoulders now. "Sweetie~" I cooed in her ears. Amy stifled a laugh and covered her mouth. I grinned at her; I was winning this battle. "Come on, Ames~" I whispered. "Don't be mad~" I smiled and kissed her.

Amy blushed and pushed her ears back. "Don't ignore me, Ames. You know you can't ignore me. I'm the blue blur, the hero of your dreams." I knew Amy's face was as red as a tomato. Amy covered her entire face, but I could see part of her cheeks. "You gonna talk to me now? You gonna tell me what I did?" I kissed her cheeks, and she removed her hands.

"Well?" I raised an eyebrow at her. Amy was so embarrassed and red-faced she couldn't talk properly. "Amy, breath in and out." I demonstrated, and she giggled at me but joined in

"Ok, ok, I'm good now..." Amy took in a deep breath. "I was never mad at you; I just wanted to see how you'd react." My shoulders slumped. "Wait. What? I thought you were mad at me! I thought I did something terrible!"

Amy laughed and patted my back. "Aww! Sweetie! You know I could never hate you!" I rolled my eyes grinned. "Sur-r-r-e!!!" I said to her. Amy kissed me, then laid down. "Night, sweetie." She said. "Night, Ames," I said and laid down next to her.

Picture Perfect

"Look what I found!" Anne called from the attic. "What is it, sweetie?" I asked her. Anne slowly climbed out of the attic and handed me an old picture.

"What's this?" I blew off some dust and gasped. "Sonic! Sonic, get in here!" I yelled at him. Loud stomps came running down the hallway to me. "What's wrong? Who's hurt?!" He asked loudly. "No ones hurt, but look what Anne found!" I showed him the picture, and he cocked his head to the side.

"It's a picture of us. So what? We have tons." He said in confusion. "What?! You don't remember this day?!" I gasped at him. Sonic shrugged, but when he saw my hurt expression, his own expression changed.

"I-I mean... Of course, I remember! That was the day we..." I narrowed my eyes at him and tapped my foot. Anne, who was clinging to my hip, narrowed her eyes as well. "Daddy, you shouldn't lie to Mommy. When Flash lied to Mommy, he gets in trouble. You don't wanna get in trouble with Mommy."

"Ain't that the truth..." I heard him whisper.

I continued my glare at Sonic as he tried to figure out a way out of this. "It was the day we... Uh... Had our first kiss?" I rolled my eyes at him. "Ugh! Men! It was the day you got me a very special present." I told him, hoping it would be enough of a clue.

"Oh! Yeah! I got you that... Thing." He grinned. I sighed at him. "Whatever... Come on, Anne, let's go play with your dolls." I smiled at her. Anne smiled a big open-mouthed grin. "Yay!"

"Wait! Ames, come back! I'm sorry, I forgot!" He called behind me.

"One second, Anne. Mommy has to talk to Daddy."

"Okay. Good luck, Dad!"

I turned around and faced Sonic. I could see in his eyes he wished he had a better memory. He gulped as I got nose to nose with him. "A-Ames?" He blushed and said my name, nervously.

"That day was the first time you ever showed the slightest interest in me. It was the day we talked about certain things. It was the day you got me a very special seashell jewelry set."

Sonic nodded. "Oh! I-I remember now! I promise!" I raised an eyebrow at him. "I swear, Ames. It was pretty pale pink seashells. We talked about how we liked each other, but we never said we loved each other. Then I got you that ice cream, and we shared it together when the others left."

I kept my eyes narrowed as I backed up. "Mommy! You coming?!" Anne called.

"On my way!" I called back and left Sonic in the hallway.

Mad? At Me?!

"Ugh! I can't believe you told the kids that!" Amy hissed at me. We were on our porch outside. "Come on, Ames! You know I didn't mean anything by it." I cupped her head in my hands, but Amy tried to push me away. She didn't have much success, so I began to kiss her.

It was my way of a desperate attempt for her to forgive me. "No! You've scarred our babies!" She spat angrily. "No, I didn't! They didn't even understand what I said!" I told her. Amy rolled her eyes.

•Flashback•

"-And then your father got me ice cream, and we shared it together." Amy smiled at Flash as she showed off the picture. "Dad stole your ice cream!" Flash laughed. "It's 'stole,' Flash." Amy corrected him. "Looks like Dad enjoyed that licking that ice cream!" Anne smiled as she snuggled into her bed.

"Not the only thing I've enjoyed licking." Sonic blushed and laughed. Amy's eyes widened as the kids looked up at him in confusion. "I meant like a Popsicle or-or-" Amy slapped Sonic in the arm as he began to laugh.12

•End Flashback•

"Ugh! You don't do that to kids, Sonic!" Amy growled at me. "Their asleep, Ames! They don't know what I meant!" I laughed and hugged her. "No! Don't touch me! You've ruined our kid's fragile, innocent minds!" I knew she was joking, so I began to kiss her neck. "Come on, baby; you know you love me!" I put it at her.

Amy rolled her eyes and giggled. "I'm trying to be mad at you! Stop it!" She giggled louder. "Nu-uh! You're mine now, Ames!" I chuckled lightly and kissed her again.

"Fine! Stop it! Okay, okay, I'm not mad anymore!" She laughed as I tickled her. "Ah-ha! See? Who's the best?" I asked her. Amy shook her head and laughed out loud. "Come on, Ames, say it!"

"You're the best! Okay, you're the best! Stop!" I let her go, and she laughed more. "Ugh... Okay, let's go in. I'm too tired to be mad now." I smirked and picked her up. "Okay, let's go." I smiled and ran her to our bed.

Swimming... It isn't fun

"Can't believe I agreed to this!" I thought as Anne and Flash ran onto the beach. Amy talked me into going to the beach with the kids as "payback" for corrupting their minds. I, of course, hated the water just as much as I had as a kid.2

Actually... That's an exaggeration. I've gotten used to it, but I'm still not a big fan.

"Sonic, come on. Flash wants to play with you." Amy said and led me to the water. "Daddy's coming, Flash!" Amy told him. "Kay!" Flash hollered.

Amy walked me all over to him. "Mommy!" Anne yelled at the top of her voice. "Yes, dear?" Amy responded. "Come here, MOMMY!!"

"I'll be right back. Take care of our boy, Sonic." She added, then went to where Anne had yelled. "Hey Flash, what did you want?" I asked him. "Take me further! I wanna go out further!" Flash pleaded. I gulped and looked out to the ocean. It was so big, and the waves looked like teeth. Like they would gobble up Flash and me in a second.2

"Uh... How about we just stay here?" I asked him. Flash looked up at me in confusion and disappointment. "I'll hold on to you! I won't go away!" I bit my lip and picked up Flash. "We can't go too far out." I smiled at him. Flash clapped and put his tiny arms around my neck.

"We're doing pretty good..." I smiled, proud of myself. Flash smiled at the water and tried to reach to touch it. Then I realized the water was just above my waist. I froze and couldn't move any further. "Daddy, go further!" Flash said and kicked his legs. His toes barely reached the water.

"I think we should just go back," I told Flash and tried to take a few steps back. It was like the sand was pulling me towards. The waves would pull back, and I felt like I was further than I was two seconds ago.

"But-"

"No buts, Flash. We have to go back." I told him sternly.

Flash sighed, obviously not happy with what I said. "Don't be sad; Mommy will take you while I'm with Anne," I told him. Flash still looked disappointed but managed a smile.

"Alright, let's go back to the shore." I slowly turned around and made my way to the sand.

***

•Later•

"It's okay, Daddy. I don't think the water is fun, either." Anne said and made a sandcastle. "It hurts when it gets in your eyes." She explained. "Yeah, I agree with you, Princess." I smiled and rubbed her head. "Hehe! Thanks, Daddy!"

Nothing Suspicious is Going On, I Promise

The next morning, Celia was the last one left in the room; everyone had gone down to breakfast without her. She didn't hear the door open as Señora entered the room.

"Celia," Señora greeted her. Celia stopped what she was doing and looked at the older woman. "Can I speak to you for a moment?"

Celia froze. After a while, she realized that she wasn't frozen, but Señora was. She looked around her and found her guardian angel sitting by the window.

"Mr. Grenda, what are you doing here?" She asked him.

He didn't answer her for a while as he stared at Señora. Celia couldn't tell what he was thinking.

"Be careful," he finally told her.

"What do you mean?" She frowned.

"Your idea is right and wrong; think about it more, but don't overthink it," he told her.

"What do you mean?" She asked her guardian, angel. "Is Señora trying to kill Mr. Powell? What should I do?"

"You did what you thought was right before, so hopefully you'll be right again," he said. Time unfroze, and Celia looked back at the waiting Señora.

"Uh, I'm kinda hungry right now, so can we talk later?" She asked. Señora nodded and left the room. Celia sighed and made her way down to the dining room.

"Did you guys know that Mr. Grenda has a child?" Dawson asked the Powells at breakfast that morning. They nodded.

"Who is it?" Emma inquired.

"That's not our secret to tell," Mr. Powell said as he dipped his spoon into his cereal.

Nobody noticed that Celia pushed her food around her plate and didn't eat any of it.

"So, how are you guys liking being King and Queen?" Harmon asked the Powells conversationally.

"It's nice," Mr. Powell answered. Señora nodded.

"Who do you think better at it?" She questioned them. Dawson nudged her and gave her a look.

"We work as a team," Señora said. She stood and pushed her chair in. "I'm going to go see what our dog is doing."

Mr. Powell watched as she left then went back to eating his cereal. The other twelve quietly watched him.

"How was your drink last night at dinner, Mr. Powell?" Celia questioned him suddenly. He looked up from his cereal.

"It was alright," he said.

"Did it taste weird at all?"

"No, why?"

"No reason."

One by one, the thirteen at the table finished their breakfasts. Nolan drifted up from his seat, and Alex followed him. They went in the direction of the game room.

Brock, Harmon, Annika, and Emma went back to the room to hang out while Dawson, Taylor, and Rachel went to find a music room. Celia and Emily went outside to catch Pokémon and Mars went down to the dungeons to visit an old friend.

Why Can't Anyone Remember That Nolan Is Dead

Just like Celia that morning, Nolan and Alex didn't notice the door of the game room open. Señora entered and closed the door behind her.

"Oh, hi, Señora," Alex greeted when he noticed her.

"Hey," Nolan greeted, glancing up from the screen.

"Can you two help me with something?" She asked them. Alex paused the game and looked at her.

"Sure."

"You can't tell anyone else about it," she told them.

"What is it?" Alex questioned.

"Wait, do you want us to help you kill Mr. Powell?" Nolan asked her. Señora didn't answer.

"Wait, really?" Alex gasped. Señora kept silent.

"We don't have to kill him," Señora tried to soften what Nolan said. "But I want to get rid of him."

"Why?" Alex asked her. Señora shrugged.

"I'm getting bored, and he's getting old. It was bound to happen sometime," she answered.

"I don't know if I can help you with that, Señora," Alex told her. Señora shrugged.

"Then I might have to kill you," she said casually.

"You can't kill me; I'm already dead," Nolan said to her. He unpaused the game and continued playing.

"Think about it," Señora said to Alex. She got up to leave and looked back at him. "But don't mention this to anyone else."

Alex sat in stunned silence as Señora left.

"Alex, come on, this mine won't mine itself."

Celia's Not The Only Killer In This House

That night at dinner, everyone had been met with either Señora or Mr. Powell. Everyone but Mars that is.

"Wait, where's Mars?" Annika questioned.

"He probably left," Brock told her as he stabbed a piece of broccoli with his fork.

"But Kim's still outside," Emily said. Brock shrugged as he shoveled the broccoli into his mouth.

Dinner was quiet that night, sides were chosen, and choices were made.

Señora presented them all with fortune cookies, which they happily opened. But upon opening theirs, Dawson, Taylor, and Rachel grew confused. Instead of a fortune, they only got a time and place. They looked up at Señora, and she gave them a look. They nodded and ate their dinner.

The next morning, Dawson, Taylor, and Rachel met Señora in a room next to the game room.

"You all agreed to help me, and I have one task for you to prove your loyalty," she said to them as they entered. They sat down uneasily as she continued. "I spoke to Alex and Nolan yesterday, and they didn't agree to help me. They already know too much. I need you three to kill them."

"What!?" Dawson gasped.

"But Nolan's already dead," Rachel said.

"Just get rid of him, I don't care," Señora said. "I don't want to see them breathing by the time the others wake up." With those words said, she promptly left the room.

"Did Señora really just ask us to kill Alex and Nolan?" Rachel asked Taylor and Dawson. They nodded. "How could she?"

"Well, she is trying to kill her husband," Dawson reminded her. Rachel sighed.

"We could stab them," Taylor suggested. "Or suffocate them. There's a window we could push them out of."

"Taylor," Dawson nervously laughed.

"What?" She retaliated. "We're her stage managers; we're required by contract to do what she asks us to do."

"But you're a minor; it's not legal if you're a minor," Dawson reminded her.

"But she wrote it into the contract. I helped her write it," she confessed. Dawson gasped.

"But I didn't sign a contract," Rachel said. "So, I don't have to do it."

"But if you don't, she's going to have you killed too," Taylor said.

"We can give them poison," Dawson suggested. "I'm pretty sure Celia carries some around for an emergency."

"But how are we going to kill Nolan?" Rachel asked.

"Vacuum."

Mars is a Weird Name

Taylor, Dawson, and Rachel crept back into the room they shared with their friends just as they began to wake. Nobody suspected a thing as they got ready for the day.

At breakfast, Señora noticed Alex and Nolan's empty seats and gave the trio an approving nod.

"Hey guys, does anyone know where Nolan is?" Celia asked her friends that night as they got ready for bed. "He hasn't haunted me all day." Nobody knew where he was.

"And does anyone know where Mars is?" Brock questioned. "I have no one to spoon now."

"You can join us," Harmon suggested from next to Emma and Annika. Brock shrugged and joined them.

"Has anyone noticed something weird going on with Taylor, Dawson, and Rachel lately?" Emma questioned Annika, Harmon, Brock, Emily, and Celia a couple of days later.

"Maybe they're working with Señora," Emily joked. Celia gasped. "Maybe," she repeated. "Because we're working with Mr. Powell.

"Shh," Brock shushed her. "Don't say it too loud, or someone will hear."

"You're just paranoid, Brock," Emma told him.

"Hey, the last time Celia was paranoid, Sharon tried to kill Jeff," he reminded her. "And have you guys noticed that Alex and Nolan hadn't been around lately?"

"Maybe they're dead," Emily joked.

"But Nolan's already dead," Annika said.

"I'm sure he could find a way to die again," Celia said. Everyone agreed.

That night at dinner, something didn't seem right. Nobody touched their foods, and nobody talked.

It was at that moment that Celia realized that everyone was frozen.

Her guardian angel burst through the doors in a frenzy.

"Celia!" He yelled. She stood in confusion. He rushed to her and gripped her shoulders. "You have to get out of here!"

"What? Why?" She asked him.

"There's no time to explain!" He told her.

"Time isn't real," she said. Mr. Grenda laughed.

"You're right," he sat down in Mars' empty seat as Celia sat in hers. "Something big is going to happen right after I leave," he told her.

"What?"

"I can't tell you."

"Why not? I'm going to know right after you leave, anyway," she protested. Mr. Grenda sighed.

"Mars and Nathan," he began. Celia gasped. "They are going to try and kill you all, and you have to leave," he pressed.

"How do you know this?"

"Because I was there." Mr. Grenda disappeared, and Mars and Nathan burst through the same doors Mr. Grenda had moments earlier. Celia stood and grabbed a butter knife as everyone else sat in confusion.

"What's happening?" Emma asked.

"Nathan?" Brock asked as he stood. "Mars?"

"I should be King," Nathan announced in a loud voice. He walked towards the Powells. The couple couldn't move out of fear because Mars was aiming an arrow at them. "Not these two. And definitely not Celia." Nathan shifted his eyes to look at Celia.

Nathan swiftly sliced the throats of the Powells. They fell forward, and everyone rose from their seats in a panic.

"You can't become King like this," Dawson said frantically to Nathan. Nathan smiled.

"Can't I?" He threw a knife, and it pierced Dawson in the heart. His friends gasped as he fell backward. "Who's next?"

Brock grabbed Harmon's hand and tried to flee, but Nathan threw a nearby vase at them, causing Brock to stumble and fall out the window. Harmon was pulled down with him.

"Mars, grab Celia and take her out of the castle. I want to kill her last," Nathan ordered. Mars grabbed her arm and dragged her outside. She turned to look back and saw the whole castle on fire.

She gasped and staggered, but Mars caught her.

"How could you do this?" She asked him. He sighed and tried to keep a straight face.

Nathan strode outside casually with a sword in hand. Celia watched as he approached her and Mars.

"I want a trophy when I kill you," he leered. He slid his finger across the blade, testing the sharpness.

"Nathan, please don't do this," she tried. Nathan shook his head as Mars tightened his grip on her arms.

"Your guardian angel isn't here to save you this time," Nathan laughed.

"Bet," Mars pushed Celia behind him and snatched the sword from his friend's hand.

"Give it back to me, Mars," Nathan said.

"No," he answered. "And my name isn't Mars; that's a dumb fucking name. My name is James Grenda." Mars swung the sword and chopped Nathan's head off.

Bedtime

Laziness

This kinda happened while I was trying to take a nap.

Don't know how it came to me; my imagination just goes with the flow, XD

Well. Enjoy this short story. Bye!

Let's just say you weren't in a good mood last night. With Peach always getting kidnapped by Bowser, the King of Koopas, and Luigi and Mario spending a week on finding her and retrieving her, you were alone most of the time. You were kinda disappointed that Mario and Luigi wouldn't let you go with them; they were saying that Bowser wasn't on your level; he was higher than that. It was hard to understand them with their Italian accents, but that's what you got from what they were saying. Well, like the idiot you are, you don't like to follow the rules as a common person would. Instead, you watch Venturiantale. But you love Venturian anyway, and you stick with watching their hilarious videos. Mostly Jordan's An Oblivion Tale series. You would laugh your butt off every time you watch Venturian; they were like you, weird and funny.

Sometimes you would wish they were your siblings! But they aren't, sadly.

But now, back to the 'I don't like common rules' thing. Mario and Luigi are at it hunting for Princess Peach, as usual. So you decided to do the dastardly, and that 'genius' idea just had to come true. Sneak into Bowser's castle. Most people would say you were crazy, but in your mind, something was telling you Bowser isn't really a bad guy. Yea, he has a dark vibe, and he breathes fire, but is he really all that bad? You can remember the times Mario had created a party with Toad, Yoshi, Peach, Daisy, Wario, and his other friends, but never invited Bowser. You felt bad for the big dragon, turtle, thing; maybe the reason he was crashing the party like a 'buzzkill' was that he was never invited to any of the parties! Maybe Mario was the buzzkill the whole entire time! You laughed a little. This reminded you of the movie 'Wreck-It Ralph.' Where Ralph tried to prove that he can be a good guy, and tried to get a medal, and met Vanellope Von Schweets in Sugar Rush. Maybe you would be Vanellope and help Bowser prove? You wouldn't be sure. But you were going to Bowser's castle, even if it kills you.

And here you are, walking out the door like the idiot you are.

You weren't sure why you were doing this; maybe you just wanted to see Bowser for once; Mario or Luigi wouldn't let you see him, so you had high attempts to finally see what the dragon looked like.

Wait, what does Bowser look like? All Mario told you was that he had a spiked shell and breathed fire. You predicted that he was a turtle, dragon thing. You play a lot of video games, like Skyrim. A turtle, dragon thing wouldn't be a surprise to you, but you really wanted to see what this thing looked like up close; maybe it's like meeting a real dragon? Was Bowser even a dragon? You suddenly skitted to a halt and smelt something burning. Ashes? Were you in Darkland now? You looked up. A gigantic castle made of stone and had Bowsers face implanted on them. Yep, this is it. You went to open the doors but then remembered.

Wouldn't Bowser have Peach locked up in here? Would you actually save Peach this time instead of Mario and Luigi? You smiled brightly at the thought. And opened the doors.

You had slightly forgotten that it would take a long time to go up to the top of the tower, and you stopped a few times to catch a breath. Then they had to fight a few Goombas. Let's say you were tired.

Very tired.

As soon as you got up to the top, you literally faceplanted with Peach staring at you with a shocked expression. You raised your hand and did a thumbs up before almost literally blacking out. You were breathing quite heavily and holding your heart. You thought you were going to have a heat stroke. Is there no AC here? Like, at all?

"Quick, he is gone now, but he will come back! Hide somewhere, anywhere!"

You literally never get a break, do you?

"Alright, just let me catch my breath, Peach."

"There is no catching breaths! You must hide before you get hurt!"

You groaned and went sluggishly up the stairs to some bedrooms. And planted on a bed, you wanted to go to sleep. You didn't care if Bowser found you. You just hope he wouldn't burn you to a crisp instead of letting you sleep. The dark met you so suddenly.

You opened your eyes and was met with an angry Bowser on top of you.

You almost faceplanted onto the floor, but he was holding you down. He had a cold stare, colder than death. Of course, he was 'Dry Bowser', once.

"Get up." He said so suddenly, and you shared the same cold stare.

"And why should I? I'm still a sleepy dragon, turtle thing! I had to climb 10,000 steps to get to the top! So don't judge me!"

Bowser still had a cold stare, but that dark vibe wasn't coming off him anymore. Was he confused?

"It doesn't make me tired."

Your eyes went wide than normal.

"Of course, it doesn't work for you! You aren't human; you're a dragon!"

Bowser looked down at you before sniffing black smoke out of his nostrils as a dragon does. You coughed, then sneezed.

"See? A dragon." You said coldly and tried to push him off you. Of course, you failed. It's 3,000 pounds!

Bowser began to laugh. What was he laughing about?

"I am no dragon. Well, maybe, I am. I don't know exactly."

Doesn't Bowser know what he is? That's a little strange.

"Um, could you get off me now? Your kinda heavy."

He then planted into you like a little puppy, almost squishing you

"What the heck?"

"Your comfy." He said, muffled from the bedsheets.

"Yep, I'm comfy; get off me, please!"

Bowser shook his head and dug deeper into you. You groaned.

"Ok, seriously."

He shushed you by putting a clawed finger on your mouth, and his breathing became shallow; he was sleeping and squishing you at the same time. There was nothing to do now, and little did you know he wasn't trying squish you; he was trying to cuddle an unknown stranger. What. The. Heck.

His tail straddled from side to side peacefully as he snored silently, but enough that you could hear it. He then grabbed you and pulled you against him, not hard, but with little force. He was warm. Like, 'even though he's a dragon lizard thing he's still warm,' kinda warm. You sighed and dug your head into the crook of his neck, and peacefully went to sleep with him. Who knew a big brute like him would have such a love for an unknown person? Or maybe he knew you and never got to see you, just like you never got to see him.

--

I had fun with this. And the title is a little misleading and had absolutely nothing to do with the story. XD

But I still had fun, and this is my first time writing Bowser; I hope he wasn't too out of character.

I was thinking of adding some of the different characters like Bowser Jr, but I couldn't think of where to put him, so I didn't add him.

Also, don't worry. Peach was saved by Mario and Luigi.

I hope you enjoyed it!

Board Games

You laughed as Bowser rolled into onto you, sniffing your hair and digging his face into your neck, biting softly.

Just a few weeks ago, you decided that you should live with the King of Koopas himself since Mario Bros. wanted to be a little picky with who you date. It was also when of figured out the Koopa had his own children.

Eight of them.

You didn't realize he had so many kids or any kids at all! What hatched them? Himself? You remember being all weird around him, and that one time he almost literally snuggled you to death. You also remember the smell of ashes always filling your nose when you walked one step into Dark Land. Always made you want to puke, but you've gotten used to it by now. Mario also started inviting Bowser to Mario Kart and even parties! He would come home sometimes bragging to his kids and you that he had won and got a golden trophy. The kids even made a trophy case for it.

The kids? They can be cute sometimes but can be a handful. Your favorite has to be Ludwig. He behaves and is very kind; he tries to stop his siblings from doing bad and tries not to give you a hard time. He also has puffy hair. Who doesn't want that?

You got off the bed and opened the drawer, taking out Candy Land. A long time favorite. You used to play this back at 3rd Base in fourth and fifth grade. Ah, the memories!

Bowser looked at you with a tilted expression, and you sighed. You pointed at the game in your hands.

"This is Candy Land. You play and try to find King Kandy! Although it's been a long time, and the game might take a while. There can only be 2-4 players, but all the kids can play!"

He looked confused but quickly nodded as he ran out to tell the kids. You went downstairs, got some chips and dip, and some soda—enough for all the kids, including you and Bowser. Tiny pitter-patters alerted you that all the Koopalings were coming down the stairs. You quickly set out the game and the chips. Just as soon as you finished, all the kids sat down around the table, Ludwig being beside you. Bowser sat beside you and smiled awkwardly. He's obviously hasn't had this kind of affection before. You giggled quietly, and Bowser blushed awkwardly. Roy gagged while Ludwig smiled. Suddenly, Lemmy jumped into your lap.

"Hey (Your Name)! Do you like King Dad?"

Both you and Bowser blushed, and Lemmy laughed.

"I knew it! (Your Name) and Bowser sitting in a tree, K-I-S-S-I-N-G!"

Roy gagged. "Lemmy, stop talkin' bout it! It's nasty!" Lemmy looked at Roy and stuck his tongue out.

You turned to Bowser and smirked, ignoring the kids. He looked at you and shrugged. You giggled and turned your attention to the kids, gaining their attention by clearing your throat.

All the kids looked at you as you smirked.

"Actually, Lemmy," you said, grabbed Bowser's chin and bringing him down to your level. "I do love him." You said as you pushed your lips against his. Roy gagged as Ludwig squealed on the inside. When you finished, Bowser picked you up and ran to his room.

Let's say the night wasn't as quiet as the Koopalings thought it to be.

Lemon!

You were melting.

I was literally melting.

Ever since you had finished the board game with the King of Koopas himself, he brought you into his room. And it was very warm. Not warm, HOT. It was like his room was filled with lava! You were like the Wicked Witch of The West from The Wizard of Oz.

"Father," a voice echoed from outside the iron door; you remembered that German accent. Bowser groaned and laid on a table, chin in hand. "What is it, Ludwig?" He asked it was responded quickly with a thick, real, German accent. "If you are planning to do, "the thing," he quoted, "be sure to use protection. Please." The room was silent as Bowser looked at you.

~LEMON AHEAD, YOU HAVE BEEN WARNED~

He grinned as he pulled a potion out from his desk and opened it. You looked at him curiously. "What's that?" You asked, blinded by the hotness. He smirked once again and drank it quickly. He groaned as he fell down on his chair, and you immediately ran up to him. "Are you ok?" You asked, worried that he had almost killed himself. But right before your eyes, he had turned into a puff of smoke. You closed your eyes and cleared the smoke in front of your eyes, and looked around.

"Bowser?" You asked, looking around. But saw nothing. Something firmly grabbed your hair and pulled your head down. You tried to shriek but realized your mouth was around something. You looked up but was quickly interrupted by thrusting in your mouth. You groaned as a slimy substance went down your throat; you quickly moved back and wiped your mouth. You were about to say something, but you found yourself sitting on a lap, hands behind your back.

"Is this rape?" You questioned, but you groaned when you felt something jab your insides. Then it hit you.

You were having sex with a random stranger. When you had time to look at him, you realized the red hair. You tried to pull back, but you were strained. "Let me, too, now. Bowser." You said sternly, but he didn't comply. Instead, he trusted something inside you.

You shrieked as it ripped your insides, and it hurt very badly.

So bad you wanted to literally cry. Then, tears came out of your eyes. It hurt so much you couldn't take it! Then, you calmed down as the pain subsided, and a calming voice whispered sweet love words into your ear and strokes your hair slowly. You tried moving around and moaned a little too loudly for comfort. "You can move now." You answered quietly, and he nodded. He began to thrust slowly into you. You grabbed his back as the pleasure almost because unbearable to not moan. You grabbed his back; he began to thrust harder. That's when you lost it.

You don't remember much from that night, only that you're sperm free. And you're pretty sure the Koopa Kids didn't spend a lot of time sleeping.8

And your pretty sure Ludwig jerked to it.

A Martian Trip

Have you ever wondered what it was like to be from mars?

I do; I am Princess Kintareen, I am the princess of mars, and I am 567 years old.6

Some humans come here, but we came to earth as well, just to prove our existence.

Have you ever wondered why asteroids land on earth?

That's because asteroids are our spaceships, or as we'd like to call it, 'asteroid ships.'

I've always wondered how humans looked like.

What is their skin color?2

Eye color?1

Their hair color.1

Humans are complicated creatures; they have never seen any of us before. To them, Martians aren't real.

Anyway, today is a big day. Today, we will be landing on earth! But, sadly, by 'we,' I mean our astronauts. My parents will never let me go there; they kept saying it was too dangerous.

But I had a plan...

Everyone cheered as our bravest of astronauts walked towards their asteroid ship. Before they could go inside the asteroid ship, I turned smaller and walked right into the ship first.

We Martians can turn smaller, to about any size we want to, for the fact.

Once we finished the countdown, we blasted to earth. The asteroid shook and shook as we blasted off. Once we landed, or rather crashed, on earth, I exited the ship and shape-shifted into a regular teenage girl.

Be careful; you wouldn't know if your best friend is a martian as well. There are 4 signs that show people aren't people.

One; we don't eat human food.2

Two; if there's a new bunch of words in the dictionary, we probably don't know them.

Three; we are probably more high-tech than the human race.

Four; rain vaporizes us, so we stay away from the rain—bad rain, rain bad.

If you know someone who fits into the list above, they're probably Martians too.

Anyway, I walked around the human town, looking around from place to place. There was more color here than I've ever thought there were. But once I came around a greenie place, there was a sign right in front of it; it read: 'Town Lake.'

It looked beautiful! The water was so clear that I could see my reflection! Except instead of seeing a regular teenage girl, I saw me; Kintareen, the martian princess. I never knew we could see our true selves when we look at our reflection.1

Soon, it was starting to get dark, and I was getting very worried, so I ran back to where we once landed. And... it wasn't there!

Oh no!

I need to get home! I shouldn't have come here in the first place! I should have listened to my parents!

So... I did the thing people did when they were homeless; I wandered around the streets like there was no tomorrow.

But there probably wasn't a tomorrow for me anyway.

Soon, it began to rain! So I ran and ran, finding a small bench... with a roof over it! I quickly rushed there and immediately took a seat there. Having nothing to do, I examined my burns.

Water burns us, just like fire burns humans. See how different our lives are?

"Hey, are you lost?" a voice calls.

Is that voice talking to me? I looked around, and I was the only person on this street.

I turned to look at who spoke to me, and I found myself face to face with a human... boy.

"Yeah, I kind of am."

"You aren't from here, are you?" the boy took a seat beside me on the bench.

"You could say that." I smile at him.

"Need a place to stay?"

"Yes!" I cried, "Please!"

"Sure." He looked at me, examining my features, "What's your name, princess?"

Princess? Does he know that I am the princess of mars?!

I had to make up a name...

Let's see...

My name is Kintareen.

What name should I go with?

Cynthia?

Tareen?

Tara?

I'll go with "Cinthia."

"Cool name." he gave me a boyish smile, "My name's Kevin."

"I've never heard of a name like that before." I thought aloud.1

Martians have never spoken with humans before... even if we could shape-shift into looking like them.

"Really?" he asks, "A lot of people have-never mind, I forgot you aren't from here."

"Okay..."

"Hey, are you okay?" he asks me, "You look like you've just escaped a fire."

"That's because... I... I did." I lie.

"Okay...?," he looks at me questioningly, "What do you do for a living?"

"Umm... work?" Why on mars did I say that?

"Okay..." he chuckles, "You're very different."

"I know..."

"C'mon." he stands up, expecting me to come with him. "I'll give ya a place to stay for the night."

"No, thank you." I look at the pouring rain, "I'll just find another place."

"What?" Kevin asks, "Are you afraid of the rain?"

"You could say that."

"Don't be. Besides, I think it'll help those burns."

It's what caused the burns, you human! "I'll just wait for the rain to stop."

"You could always use my umbrella."

"Umbrella?"

"You don't know what an umbrella is?"

"Nope," Hey, don't judge! It doesn't rain on mars, so we don't need this umbrella thing.

"You don't get out much, do you?"

"Nope." I gotta stop lying.

"Here." He opened the umbrella and placed it under the rain. "See? The rain won't touch ya."

He was right. It was like a rain protection thing! I should teach this to my people when I get home if I get home.

We headed to his house, where he allowed me to use the guest room.

Kevin surprisingly lived by himself... in such a big house.

As we ate dinner, I asked him, "Why do you live by yourself?" I bluntly ask, "You look a bit young to live by yourself."

"You're too young to be roaming the streets alone." He smirks.

I'm 567 years old, you human! "Good point."

Once we finished eating dinner, we went our separate ways and went to sleep.

Weeks went by, and Kevin took me in as if I was his own. He has even opened up to me.

Wanna know why he lives by himself?

His family died, in a fire, when he was little. Poor kid. He was also willing to help me that night because he knew how I felt. His house burned down during the fire. So he practically roamed the streets, too, looking for shelter.

I feel pretty guilty that I haven't told him my secret, so I decided to tell him, even if it may be against the law.

"Kevin?"

"Yeah?"

"I need to tell you something..."

"What is it, Cinthia?"

A shiver ran down my spine when he said my name, even if it wasn't my real name. For the past week, I think I feel a strong affection towards Kevin. In human words, I liked him.

"I'm not what you think I am."

"What are you---"

"I'm a martian from mars."

I expected him to scream or to tell me to leave his house and check-in in a mental hospital, but now, he didn't... he laughed!

"Martian?" he repeats, "Seriously, Cinthia, from all the jokes you could come up with, you chose that?"

"I'm not joking." I use a serious tone.

Before he could speak, I shape-shifted back into... me.

My tan human skin turned into my red one, my blue eyes turned back into my green ones, and my black hair shifted back into my dark red hair.

"Oh my!" he took a deep breath, "You weren't joking."

"I know... you can freak out if you want."

"Nah, I'm good." He assures me, "So... you're a---"

"And my real name is 'Kintareena.'" I admit, "But if you want, you could still call me 'Kinthia.'"

"Okay, but---"

"I need your help."

"You wanna get home, don't you?"

"Are you kidding?" I ask, "I want to stay here, with you, forever!" I practically yelled at him, "But, I'm not just a regular martian, I'm a martian princess."

"Oh... so... you gotta get home?"

"Yes?"

"I'll help you." he says, "I could be able to sneak you inside a space station. You do know how to drive a spaceship, right?"

"We don't have spaceships on mars, but we have asteroid ships. They're practically the same thing, I think."

"Okay..." he trails off. "Let's sneak you in."1

Sooner or later, I was in front of a big spaceship, ready for blast-off.

I looked at Kevin through one of the spaceship windows as the spaceship counted down.

Five...

I still can't believe that this guy was willing to help a homeless person in the middle of the night... a complete stranger for the matter...

Four...

I might have been missing for weeks... but I seriously don't regret it. I wasn't going to forget Kevin either.

Three...

I've never expected humans to be so sweet. Growing up, I imagined humans taking over mars. But Kevin proved me wrong. He was one of the most caring people I know.

Two...

But we could never be together... it just wasn't possible.

One...

The spaceship took off.

And I sent Kevin a message with my mind.

'I love you.'

I know he couldn't reply, but I just couldn't bear to hear him say he didn't love me back.

A martian fell for a human.

But a human can never love a martian.

TV Addict

I've been watching TV all my life. Even when I'm supposed to be sleeping, I watch TV.

My parents say I should get out more; that I'm always just sitting around, watching some movie. They say it's a bad thing, but I don't see why it is.

One night, I was watching my favorite movie on TV when my mom called from the kitchen, "Charles!"

"Yeah?"

"Go to bed; it's passed your bedtime."

"Okay."

I turned off the TV and head upstairs to my room. Once I was there, I turned off my lights and turned on my laptop. I watched another one of my favorite movies, a horror film, to be exact.

In the middle of watching the movie, it froze.

"C'mon!" I groan.

In a split second, I was sucked inside the movie. Oh shit!1

This movie was about a guy who entered a haunted house. Damn it!

I've never thought that this movie was scary, but now that I'm here, I'm very, very scared!

This is the part where the dude screams, because a zombie came out of the cabinet, "AHHHHHHHH!"

Right on cue.

The kid ran upstairs, a big mistake.

I, on the other hand, had to find a way out of here.

I turned around and came face to face with a lady.

Not just any lady.

A monster!

The lady's hair was messy, some of it standing as she got electrocuted. Her eyes were very wide and red! She had long, boney fingers!

"You---" she croaked as she walked closer to me.

"AHHHH!" I screamed and ran the other way.

I entered another room... a big mistake.

There were a bunch of witches who were ripping the kid's organs out. SICK!

"Your turn!" one of them grabbed me, and they placed me on a table. One of them was holding my hands; one of them was holding my legs as the others prepared to rip open my skin.

"AHHHHH!" I scram.

And stood up from the bed.

It was a dream!

Thank the heavens!

Lesson learned; I will never watch that much TV again!

Ever since that dream, I started going out more and limited my time on watching TV, and I stopped watching horror films.

The Shell

I am Lacy; I am a 6-year-old girl.

I have a shell; it was the prettiest shell in the world, to me, at least.

I got it a few years back; my family and I went to the beach on a fine spring day because we were invited to my friend's birthday party. My friends and I were playing in the ocean, and that's when I found the shell. From then on, I brought the shell whenever I went to the beach.

And every time I went, everything went fine, as if the shell brings me good luck.

It was very pretty, so I brought it home with me after the party. It was there to remind me of that day.

Now, it was summer, the hottest of all seasons.

"Mommy, can we go to the beach?" I plead, "I'm sweating; this heat is bad!"

"Sure, sweetie, go wear your swimsuit, and we'll be on our way."

"Yay!" I shout as I ran to my room.

I wore my swimsuit and wore my normal clothes over it, and I ran back to my mom. She had already finished packing the things we needed by the time I got to her.

"Mommy, did you bring my shell?" I ask, remembering I always bring it with me.

"Yes, I did." She answers.

We got in our car, and we drove to the beach. When we arrived, I was so excited to play around that I quickly ran out of the car, with my shell and my shovel and pail set in both hands. I ran until I decided to sit. So I sat on the sand.

I placed my shell right beside me, and I started making my castle. My mommy joined me sooner or later, and we finished making the most beautiful sandcastle ever!

"Sweetie, do you want to take a dip in the ocean?" my mommy asks, "We need to wash away this sand."

"Let's swim!" I cheer.

She placed on my floaters, we wore our swimsuits, and we swam in the ocean.

"Yay!" I shout as I splashed around.

This is really the way to beat the summer heat!

Once I finished swimming, I saw a mini ice cream parlor, "Mommy, can we please buy ice cream?" I plead.

"Sure."

We walk up to the man who sold the ice cream and ordered two cones.

"Flavors?" he asks for our ice cream flavors.

"Chocolate!" I cheer.

"One chocolate and one strawberry." My mommy tells the boy.

He handed us our ice cream, and we sat on the sand, eating away.

Once we finished eating, my mommy asks me, "Lacy, do you want to go home now?"

"Yup."

"Okay."

"Can I help you pack?" I offer.

"Please."

We packed everything, but just when we were ready to head back home, I shouted, "Where's my shell?!"

I dropped whatever I was carrying and ran back to where we built the sandcastle. I looked around the castle, but it wasn't there!

I dug the sand surrounding the castle in hopes of finding the shell, but I didn't find it.

I dug and dug, but I didn't find it. Instead, my eyes caught something... a shell!

I pulled it out of the sand to see that it wasn't my shell.

I cried.

"Sweetie, it's okay," my mommy tries to comfort me, but the tears just wouldn't stop flowing.

"I can't find the shell!" I weep.

"Why don't you just keep this one instead?" she shows me the shell that I just found, "It's much prettier than the other one."[1]

It was true, the shell was prettier, "But the other one had more memories!" I argue.

"Then, we'll make new memories, okay, baby?"

I sniffled, "Okay."[1]

Once we got back home, I placed my new shell in a glass case, where I used to keep my old one. By the next morning, I was in for a surprise.

The new shell I found wasn't just a shell.

It was a crab's shell!

"Mommy!" I shout, "Look!"

She ran inside my room, "What's wrong?" she asks, "Are you hurt?"

"Look!" I point to the crab.

"I guess we have a new pet." Mommy smiles.

From then on, we took care of the crab, and I named him 'Crabie.'

I guess I was happy, after all.

The Princess And The Kidnapper

Once upon a time, there was a princess who was fairest in the land.

She was betrothed to the bravest of all princes in the land.

He was handsome, brave, and strong.

But she doesn't love him.

Nor did he love her.1

The week before their marriage, the princess took a walk around her kingdom dressed like a normal girl, with a hood over her head, so no one would recognize her.

As she walked and walked, someone grabbed her by her wrist.

The princess screamed.

The person placed her in a sack.

Soon, when they reached an abandoned house, the guy took her out of the sack.

"You do know that that hood isn't going to hide your face, right?" he smirks.

"What do you want?" she questions.

"I kidnapped you... for ransom." He smiles wickedly, "Think of all the money your parents would be willing to give for your release."

"Free me, and you shall not be thrown in the dungeons." The princess bargained.

"Nah, I'm good." The boy shrugs, "Once I get the money and set you free, I'll leave, to another land."2

"How dare you betray your princess?!"

"You're not my princess... you're his." He pointed to a shadowy figured.

The princess turned her head to look at the figure. It was her prince! Her betrothed! He was tied up in one of the chairs.

I'm never going to get out of here! The princess thought.

She thought it was the end. Her parents would pay for the ransom; she knew they'd do anything for her safety.

Weeks passed, and their parents have not yet paid for their freedom. The princess was beginning to lose hope.

One day, when she and her prince were eating their pieces of bread that the kidnapper had given them, the kidnapper walked into the room, "You have to go."

The princess nearly choked on the piece of bread that she was chewing, "What?"

"You and pretty boy here have to go."

"Did they pay the ransom?"

"They were worried sick when they found out that you two were missing," he explained, "but I never handed out the ransom."

"Why?"

"I can't explain." He unlocks the chains that tie her and the prince to the walls of the abandoned house, "You just have to go."

He sets the prince and the princess free, and they never saw the kidnaper again.

Years passed, and the prince and the princess were already happily married and had a baby girl.

Throughout these years, one question lingered in the princess's head.

Why did the kidnapper set them free?

Mindy in
Fairytale Land

Hi, my name is Mindy, and this is one of the coolest--yet freakiest--things that ever happened in my whole life:

It was pretty boring today; I was an only child, so I didn't have anyone to play with. Being an 8-year-old girl, I needed someone to play with.

I usually imagined playmates since my parents wouldn't let me out of the house on weekends since I was practically accident-prone.

I live in Paris, France. I've been living here all my life. This house was pretty old, so old, that even my ancestors used to live here.

My parents were at work, and my babysitter was pretty much asleep, so I was bored.

I decided to walk around the house; I checked the basement first. It was dusty because we haven't cleaned here in a while.

I walked up to an old bookshelf. It was dusty too.

But a story title caught my eye, 'Rapunzel'!

I loved that story! It was my favorite fairytale!

I decided to read it, I pulled the book out of the shelf, but it didn't go out all the way through. Instead, the book went back on the shelf, and the shelf moved!

It moved sideways, and behind it was a small door!

I walked up to the door. I twisted the doorknob. And I couldn't believe my eyes!

It was like a whole other land was behind the bookshelf!

My grandma told me that this house was full of magical secrets, but I never actually saw magical stuff until now...

I walk inside... it was a fairytale land!

I saw different storybook characters. I saw the gingerbread man, the three little pigs, Snow White, and so much more!

I looked around, but I didn't see Rapunzel.

So, I decided to go ask for directions; I walked up to The Old Woman (who lived in a shoe) and asked, "Excuse me, ma'am, do you know where Rapunzel is?"

"Oh my, my, you can't visit her." She explains, "She is still locked up in the tower..."

That's when I made a mental note:

'I have to save Rapunzel!'

"Do you know where her tower's located?" I ask.

"Yes... right over there." She points in a direction. "Just follow that direction until you see Humpty Dumpty; you may ask for more directions from him."

"Thank you."

I took the path where she pointed to, and soon, I saw Humpty Dumpty.

But he was falling from the wall!

I ran up to him, and luckily I made it just in time to catch him!

"Are you okay?" I ask as I placed him on the ground so that he may stand.

"I am now, thank you." he gives me a toothy smile.

"No problem..." I trail off, "Do you know the way to Rapunzel's tower?"

"Yes... right over there." He points north.

And I saw it, Rapunzel's tower... and it was pretty tall.

"Thanks. Bye!" I started walking towards the tower, "Stay away from high walls!" I call out.

"I will!" Humpty calls back.

Wow, I can't believe I saved Humpty Dumpty!

Once I reached the tower, I saw that the prince was calling out to Rapunzel.

As he climbed her hair, I thought of different ways to rescue her. Hmm.........

What if she climbed a tree down?

I looked around the tower, but no tree was near it.

What if she jumped down?

The towers pretty high; if she did jump, she would get down... but with a few broken bones.

What if she landed on something soft?

That's genius!

I looked around to find something soft, but there was nothing soft around here.

Let's see... was there any fairytale with something soft involved? Think for a while...

The Princess and the Pea!

I could borrow one mattress!

I looked around and saw one of the three pigs. I walked up to him and asked for directions.

Once I received it, I started my walk. Soon, I reached a castle.

It was beautiful!

I knocked on the front door.

A man opened the door, "Who are you?"

"I'm Mindy, and I need to see the princess."

"Right this way."

He led me to a big, big, very big room.

It turns out; the princess was already married to the prince.

"Your highness," I bow.

"Hello." She greets.

"May I borrow a mattress?"

She gives me a weird look, "A mattress?"

"Yes, please?"

"Umm... okay?"

Soon, one of the servants brought me a mattress.

It was lighter than I thought...

Once I was back at Rapunzel's tower, I called "Rapunzel!"

She looked down, "Yes?"

Wow, she was so pretty! I wish I were as pretty as her!

"Jump down!" I point at the mattress.

Once she was on the ground, she asked me, "What's your name, dear?"

"Mindy..."

"Well, Mindy..." she turns into the witch! "I will kill you!" she points a dagger at me.

"AHHHHHHH!"

I stood up from the bed.

Was it a dream?

Thank god!

But it seemed so real...

I ran back to the basement. I pulled the book out of the self.

Just like expected, the bookshelf moved, exposing the door!

The witch was real!

"AHHHHHHHHHHHHHHHHHHHH!"

And from then on, my favorite fairytale was 'The Little Mermaid.'

The Monster Under My Bed

I have always been afraid of sleeping by myself, mainly because there was a scary monster under my bed!

I have tried telling mommy that I've heard growling noises in the middle of the night, but since I was 7 years old, she told me that I just imagined things.

I suggested spending the night with mommy, but sadly, her bed was only enough for her and daddy.

Tonight was just like any other night: restless.

Those growling noises just won't stop!

I hid under my blanket, telling myself that I just imagined things.

Soon enough, the growth stopped. But before I could rejoice, two hairy hands came from under the bed... and pulled at my two feet!!!

I tugged at whatever my little hands could reach, but the monster was a zillion time stronger.

Soon, I fell off the bed, and let me tell you something; it was painful!

Once I was under the bed, I screamed at the top of my lungs, "Ahhhhhh!" only to have a hand cover my mouth.

"Shhh!"

Even if the monster was shushing me, its voice was quite scary.

I used all my strength to removed its hand from my face. "D-don't eat m-me." I stutter.

Since I mostly slept with the lights on, I could see the monster's face... and it was scary, no wait, it was frightening!

"I no eat." the monster said in a very deep voice.

"W-what?" did it just say he wouldn't eat me? More importantly, did it just talk?

"Me good," he reassures me.

"But, you're a monster..."

"No eating you." he promises, "I eat rats."

Okay, that's pretty gross, but since it said I wouldn't get eaten, I was okay with that.

Plus, I knew now that he was the reason why I haven't seen any rats around here in a while...

"Do you have a name?" I ask.

"Ree," he growled.

"Um... cool name?" I raise an eyebrow, "Why did you drag me here, Ree?"

"Me alone."

Aw, poor guy! He needed a friend.

"I'll be your friend, Ree." I smiled and extended my hand out for a shake, "I'm Trixie."

He surprisingly didn't shake back; instead, he licked my hand!

Ewwww!

Oh well, I have a new friend now!

RIP the Drama Kids

"It's too bad that Nolan and Mikayla aren't here," Señora sighed as everyone came on stage. "They would have loved this."

"What are we doing?" Emma questioned as Mr. Powell lined them up in front of a long bucket filled with water.

"Are those apples?" Alex asked as he peered inside the buckets.

"No, actually," Señora smiled mischievously. "Those are pomegranates." The drama kids groaned in despair.

"The first one to get three pomegranates wins," Mr. Powell explained. Everyone sighed as they got on their knees in front of the bucket.

"Ready....set...go!"

Mars, Brock, Cece, and Alex plunged their faces into the water. Annika, Harmon, Emily, Celia, Dawson, and Will hesitantly went in while Emma just shook her head.

Emma sighed and began to put her head in as Mars broke from the water with a pomegranate between his teeth, Celia right after him.

"One for Mars and one for Celia!" Mr. Powell announced happily.

After a while of pomegranate bobbing, Señora realized that Will wasn't moving and was sitting with his head under the water. He came up for air just as she was beginning to become worried.

"Three pomegranates!" Mr. Powell called as he grabbed Mars' arm and raised it in the air victoriously.

"Time for voting," Señora announced as Mr. Powell cleared the stage.

Señora handed out pieces of papers to everyone and told them to write down a name beside the name Mars.

The gang looked uneasily at each other, not wanting to kill their friends potentially. But they did anyway.

Mr. Powell collected their votes and put them in a bowl.

"Stand up," Señora ordered them. They stood and waited for Mr. Powell to read their names, then they could sit down in safety.

Mr. Powell read off everyone's names, but Dawson's and Will's. He stopped for a moment and looked at them.

"Dawson," he began sadly. "You may sit down."

Will was the last one standing, and later that night, he was yeeted into a volcano.

Why Am I Crying In The Club Right Now

The next morning, the remaining ten were quietly led into Señora's classroom. Emma's face was red as they sat down.

"No one can sit in the back," Señora told them as she entered the room. The ones in the back sighed and moved towards the front.

"Today," Señora began. "Mr. Powell and I will play you a series of sad vides, and the only one who does not cry will be granted immunity from tonight's votes."

"Our first video," Mr. Powell announced joyfully as he logged into YouTube. "Is a classic."

The ASPCA logo appeared on the screen, and Emma groaned.

"Sorry, Emma, " Señora laughed as Emma began to cry. She buried her face in her arms as the video began to play.

"Nobody cares about this," Emily said. "No one will cry. Besides, Emma."

The video ended, and Emma and Alex were led out of the room.

"Wait, I haven't seen this movie yet," Brock protested as Mr. Powell loaded up another video.

"Neither have I," Señora shrugged indifferently.

The end of Avengers: Infinity War began to play, and Emily laughed.

"Isn't this funny?" She laughed as Spider-Man died. "God, I'm dead inside."

After that, several more people had to leave, and even Mr. Powell had to leave at one point. Señora sighed as she shook her head and took his spot behind the computer.

Eventually, only Mars, Dawson, and Celia were left.

"Congratulations," Señora said. "You're all dead inside."

"Guess who's going to win, again," Mars boasted.

"Shut up, Mars," Celia retorted. "You won last time; it's my turn now."

After a few more videos, Dawson was proclaimed as the dead inside.

Later that night, the gang waited anxiously for the Powells to count their votes. Señora found the crown from Greek Gods, and Dawson was currently wearing it.

"Stand," Señora ordered as Mr. Powell held the cards in his hands.

Eventually, Cece and Mars were the only ones left standing.

"Cece," Mr. Powell began. "I hope you like volcanos."

Cece's face dropped as Mars quickly sat down in his seat.

"Seriously, Mr. Powell?" She asked as she stalked off towards the volcano and throwing herself in.

I Use My Heelys to Escape My Feelies

"Our next challenge for you includes you are putting something on," Señora announced the next day. Annika, Celia, Brock, Mars, Emma, Emily, and Dawson looked at each other apprehensively as Mr. Powell unveiled their new item of clothing.

"Are those Heelys?" Brock asked in awe. Señora nodded solemnly as Mr. Powell distributed the shoes.

"I already have mine on," Celia said as he went to hand her a pair. He nodded and kept them for himself.

"What's the challenge?" Annika asked Señora as they laced on their new shoes.

"The challenge is to see who goes the farthest in the Heelys," she answered.

"We get to practice with these first, right?" Emma asked. Señora shook her head.

"That's not fair," Mars said as he slowly stood up.

"Get good," Celia smirked.

"I'm going to heely off a cliff," Emily said monotonously.

"Okay, everyone, line up," the seven slowly made their way behind a solid black line, besides Annika, Celia, and Dawson, who glided over.

"Ready...set...go!" Mr. Powell called. Brock fell backward before Mr. Powell called "go," and Emma didn't move at all, afraid that she was going to fall.

Emily tried her hardest, but she veered to the left and ran into a wall. Mars made it a short distance, but he wasn't good enough.

Dawson, Celia, and Annika sped along easily as the others watched.

By the end of the race, Celia was a mile ahead of everyone else, and she was declared the winner.

Dawson, along with the Heelys, was thrown into the volcano.

Dance Break

"I hope you're all ready for a little dancing," Señora smiled the next morning. "And it's not a conga line this time." The drama kids sighed in relief.

"What is it?" Brock asked. They all suddenly noticed Mr. Powell sitting behind a DJ booth at the back of the stage.

"Line up, please," Señora told them ominously. They did as she asked and she explained that the last one dancing won.

Mr. Powell hit a button, and "Cotton Eye Joe" blasted through the speakers. Everyone groaned as Mars instantly began to dance.

The others quickly joined him, but Brock and Emily used up their stamina too quickly and had to drop out.

Celia would have pointed and laughed at them, but she was too focused on dancing.

"Cotton Eye Joe" played on loop for hours until only two remained. Celia, Emma, Emily, Brock, and cheered as Mars and Annika continued to dance.

Mars hadn't even begun to sweat when Annika dropped out.

That night, just before Mr. Powell began to read off the names, Annika had a sudden realization.

"I just lost the game," she announced out of the blue.

Everyone groaned.

"Can I have my paperback?" Emma asked the Powells. "I want to change my vote."

"Yeah, me too," Celia agreed. Brock, Emily, and Mars nodded as they changed their votes.

"Do I even have to read it?" Mr. Powell sadly asked Annika once he had the papers again.

She shook her head and quietly yeeted herself into a volcano.

Three People Eat Candy and One Dies

"I have another problem," Señora yet again announced. "I didn't have time to make a challenge."

"Señora," Emma sighed.

"So we're just going to do Eeeney Meeney Miney Moe," she told them. "It's different from when we just voted someone off."

Brock was tossed into a volcano that night.

"Now that there's only four of you left, I feel like we should play a game of Super Todo," Mr. Powell handed out the playing cards as Señora briefly explained the rules.

"Do you have prizes?" Mars questioned. Señora nodded and pulled out a bowl of candy from her cupboard.

The Super Todo board was filled with their now-dead friends' names, first and last names in separate boxes. Nolan's name was free space.

The game started, and soon enough, Celia earned a Todito, along with a piece of candy. She snacked on it as she watched Emma, Emily, and Mars try and earn a Todo.

Mars was the next to earn candy and a Todo. He plunged his hand into the bowl and pulled out every single Cowtail.

Emma and Emily continued their game, Mars, and Celia peering over their shoulders as they ate their candy.

"Why'd you put that one there?" Mars questioned Emma. "It's never going to get called."

"Shut up," Emma swatted his hand away and tried to ignore him.

The last name that Señora called was Will's.

"Super Todo!" Emma yelled.

"Wait, I have one too," Emily said after Emma grabbed a piece of candy. Señora shook her head.

"Should have called it sooner," she told her.

Emma slurped her sucker as she watched Emily be yeeted into the volcano.

Mr. Powell Doesn't Win

"This challenge is not my favourite, but at Celia's request, we will do it," Señora said the next morning.

"Wait, what is it?" Celia questioned. Señora gave her a look. "Oh, we're comparing our dick sizes."

"What?" Mars asked, appalled. He looked uncomfortably from the girls to Señora. "Are you serious?"

"Sadly," Señora sighed.

"I'm not doing that," Mars denied.

"Weak," Emma said.

"Come on, weenie, show us your weenie," Celia taunted him.

"You wish," he said before walking off in search of a volcano to meet himself into.

"Now what?" Celia questioned as Mars finally disappeared from their sight.

"I don't know," Señora shrugged carelessly. "You can fight or something."

"But that's too easy," Celia said.

"Bet," Emma glared at her.

The fight that commenced between Emma and Celia is considered to be one of the greatest battles that ever existed. A trained assassin who killed the prince of a planet against a girl who just wanted some chicken strips. Obviously, the assassin won.

That night on the steps of the volcano her friends were ruthlessly yeeted into, Celia was crowned Queen of the planet. Nolan's ghost even came to watch.

As Celia watched her new kingdom from her castle window, she felt unsettled.

"Minecraft Steve," she said, turning to look at the Minecraft Steve statue that stood gloriously in the room. "Something doesn't feel right, but it might just be the pebble in my Heelys."

Dory's Birthday

Dory's birthday is today, and Nemo and Marlin want to surprise birthday party which. With Dory, it is easy; Charlie, Jenny, Nemo's class, and Mr. Ray, along with Hank, Bailey, and Destiny, are all coming. The good thing about Dory is that she loves surprises and games, which always works. Dory has said before that she doesn't remember when she has last celebrated her birthday. Which made Marlin and Nemo very sad; they have to get things for the party and keep her distracted, so they have Bailey and Destiny do the job.

"Hey Dory, how about we go and practice whale songs!" says Destiny

"Okay!" says Dory

"Yay! Oh yeah, Happy birthday!" says them both

"Aw, you guys so sweet," says Dory

So off the three go talking only in the whale, Nemo and Marlin smile and go off to get ready for the party.

"What should we get her, Dad?" asks Nemo

"Well, we are getting her a collection of seashells as they are special to her, which I already know her parents aren't. They said that her parents are making her a better house so she could have more room than basically a bedroom. The kids will mostly get her toys and games; the same goes for Mr. Ray, not to be mean or something but to help her with her ADHD and play with her. Hank doesn't know what he is getting her; Destiny and Bailey are making her a necklace out of human things. " says Marlin

He starts collecting some pretty shells with Nemo.

"Dad, what is ADHD?" asks Nemo

"Well, that means Attention-deficit/hyperactive disorder," says Marlin

"Does that mean that there is something wrong with her?" asks Nemo, getting worried

"No, she is completely fine; anyone can live a normal life with it; it is like your lucky fin but in her brain," says Marlin

"You're confusing me, dad," says Nemo

"Basically, her brain works differently than yours, and I's does. She gets distracted easier, and some things will bore her easier. Such as remember telling you about the jellyfish incident?" asks Marlin

"Yeah, you said she named a jellyfish squishy," says Nemo, giggling at the memory

"Yeah, she did; I was trying to talk to her, and the jellyfish came to her, and that distracted her from what I was saying. She totally forgot what was happening and that some jellyfish are aggressive, especially if they feel that someone harmed one of their own. Basically, it is easy to bore her, and it is easy to distract her. " says Marlin

"Oh, okay, so it doesn't hurt her; it just makes her think differently, which isn't a bad thing. It makes her," says Nemo, happily that it won't hurt her.

"Exactly that," says Marlin

Marlin smiles, glad that Nemo is taking it so great; he was afraid that Nemo would treat Dory differently because too. However, kids don't normally see black and white, which Marlin has forgotten over the years. He then goes back to helping Nemo collect seashells for Dory. After they get done with that, they get to work on setting things up and entertaining the guests until it was time for the party. Marlin actually sees Destiny bringing her back, so he has them all hide.

"What's going on, guys?" asks Dory, excited

"You can look in 3,2, 1," says Bailey and Destiny

They uncover her eyes, and everyone pops out from their hiding places.

"Surprise! Happy Birthday, Dory!" says, everyone

"*gasps* Wow! Guys, this is amazing!" says Dory

She looked around all happy and met all her guests.

"So Dory, what do you think?" asks Nemo

"I think this is the best thing ever! Thank you. Also, what are we waiting for? Let's a party!" says Dory

So the party began, and everyone plays games and enjoys their time spending as much as they can with Dory, especially Jenny and Charlie. They even carry in her cake for her.

"Make a wish, birthday girl," they say

She smiles and thinks for a while, then blows out the candles. Everyone cheers, then it is time for gifts, which Dory loves all of them, especially the house that her parents made for her where her old house was. She notices there is a shelf in there made of coral.

"What's the shelf for?" asks Dory

"It's a surprise," says Jenny

"You just have to wait and see," says Charlie

"Ooo yay!" says Dory

After Jenny and Charlie, the final gift is from Nemo and give her the shells that they put in a box they found that was dropped in the ocean.

"Ooo look, shells! I have nowhere to put them, but I love them!" says Dory

"How about your new shelf?" suggests Nemo

"Oo good idea," says Dory

So she and Marlin put the shells there the way Dory wanted them, and then they enjoyed the rest of the party.

Kid's New Playmate and Sequal:

Nemo and his friends were enjoying some time after school while Dory and Marlin were talking to the adults, well until Dory got bored and started playing with the kids.

"She is a spunky one," says Ted, Pearl's father

"She gets bored easily, I noticed," says Bill, Tad's father

"Yes, she is," says Marlin

"Well, she looks like she is adjusting well, being she was not from here and moved in a week ago," says Bob, Sheldon's father

Sheldon sneezes, getting far away. "...His allergies are acting up again."

"Uh..yeah, as for Dory, she adjusted well. She never thought she would. Oh hey, when is the parent-teacher conference again?" asks marlin

"Soon. He said he would be back; he disappears when he sees that the kids are taken care of. He was helping Kathy get home because her mom was running late," says Bill

"Poor girl, well hopefully she gets home alright," says Marlin

"oh yeah, with Mr. Ray by her side, she will be just fine," says Ted

"Yeah, I know I trust Mr. Ray. I just meant that Kathy gets taken home a lot," says Marlin

"Yeah..." says the others

"Everyone goes home now!" says a worried Mr. Ray

They all look at him confused; it isn't like him to get worried unless the others are in danger.

"What's wrong, Mr. Ray?" asks Nemo

"Uh. I just need you to go home, Nemo, and quickly," says Mr. Ray

"Your voice says something is wrong, Mr. Ray," says Pearl

"Nothing to worry over Pearl, if you go home now," says Mr. Ray

"Mr. Ray, you never rush us home," says Sheldon, before sneezing again

He doesn't get a chance to explain as a whale makes noises.

"Ooo, a whale! I speak whale!" starts dory, he says more, and now dory gets worried, "Um...okay kids, let's get you to your dads and home now!"

"Wait! What did the whale say, Dory?" asks Tad

"Uh...well, he said he wants to swallow us," says Dory laughing nervously

That makes everyone panic and start gathering their kids; however, the whale comes and swallows Pearl, Sheldon, and Tad.

"Pearl! Sheldon! Tad!" calls the parents and Nemo

They don't know what to do.

"Oh, no...oh no. I am so sorry," says Mr. Ray

"You tried to warn them..." says the parents.

Marlin holds Nemo close and makes sure he doesn't look. The whale starts swimming and then blows them up, making Pearl, Sheldon, and Tad laugh, and everyone else looks stunned. The whale makes more sounds.

"Oh! He doesn't want to eat us. He wants to play with the kids and help make sure the kids get home safe until he has to go back home," says Dory

"H-he said all that?" says Mr. Ray

"Uh-huh, he also says he is sorry for scaring the parents," says Dory

"Uh..." says the adults

"Dad, that was so much fun!" says Pearl, Tad, and Sheldon. "Can we do it again?!"

"Um...sure?" they say, unsure

"Dad can I go too?" asks Nemo

"Be careful," says Marlin

The whale starts "talking" again.

"Oh, okay!" says Dory

"What did he say?" asks Marlin

"He will make sure the kids will get home safely. We can all go home," says Dory

The parents aren't sure but are afraid to question it. However, they don't go home; instead, they stay out of the whales and kids' eyesight, except for Dory, who starts on home to wait for Dory.

"Dory?! What are you doing?" hisses Marlin quietly

"Going home. Remember? The whale said he would take Nemo home, and I trust him; he looks like the whale who helped us get to Sydney. Ooo! I remembered something else." says Dory, excited

"You expect us to go home when he has the kids?!" asks Ted, baffled

"Well yeah. I trust the whale, and I don't want Nemo to be home alone, so off I go. Marlin, your welcome to join me." says Dory; she goes straight home.

The kids, not even paying attention to the parents, continue to play with the whale.

"This is so much fun," says Nemo

"Have you tried using his tongue as a slide, Nemo?" asks Pearl

"No. but I want to," says Nemo

"Let's go then!" says Tad

"Yeah, come on, Nemo!" says Sheldon

Nemo looks and doesn't see his dad, so he finds that as a trust thing and goes with the trio in the whale. They wait their turn and then slide down the tongue together, laughing the whole way; they get sprouted out of the whale's hole on the top like Marlin and Dory did in the past while looking for love the whole thing, and the others decide to slide down just like Nemo and his friends do before him. They do this a few times until they get tired and let the whale know.

In the meantime, the parents shake their heads and turn back to their kids to see them gone and the whale swimming off slowly; they panic and start following the whale to the Great Barrier Reef. The whale stops at Pearl's home and drops her off. The parents are baffled; Ted goes over to her and hugs her. The others let him be with his daughter and follow the whale as more children get dropped off. Finally, they make it to Sheldon's home where Bob hugs him, then to Tad's home where Bill hugs Tad. The more kids get dropped off, the more the parents relax, finding the whale less threatening and more of a good thing. Finally, Nemo gets home, where he is greeted by Dory.

"That was so much fun, Dory. Oh! *to the whale* Thank you, Mr. Whale, for taking me home!" says Nemo

"Oh cool I am glad you had fun, Nemo," says Dory

"I did; where is dad?" asks Nemo

"Um, not sure," says Dory

"I am right here," says Marin, smiling. "I am sorry, Dory, I should have trusted you."

"That's okay; about what?" asks Dory

"Err, never mind, let's just go inside," says Marlin

They smile and head in; the next day, the whale returned, and this time the parents went home to let the kids play with their new friend. They now knew that the whale would not hurt the kids and would transport them home when they got home. This went on for a few days; the whale would come to play with the kids and then go home. However, one day, the whale turned to the parents first and started talking again.

"Uh, Dory?" asks Mr. Ray

"He said he couldn't take the kids home today. He has to go home, but he will play with them until they are tired. And say bye to the kids," says Dory

He talks again, knowing the kids will want his attention soon.

"He also said that he hopes to come back again," says Dory

The parent's smile, and all agree, telling marlin, marlin agrees too.

"Yeah, we would like that," says Marlin

Dory translates that to him, and the whale smiles and plays with the kids until he has to go. It is a wonderful time for everyone, but the kids aren't too happy about their friend having to leave. But are happy to hear he will be back again one day.

It has been a couple of years since the kids have had a playdate with the whale. Bailey, Destiny, and Hank are all busy today adjusting to their homes outside of the reef. The others decide to help them out with that since they will be visiting them a lot. As it is too much to ask them to come all the way to the reef and go back will be their permanent living area for all of the whales.

"We have to talk to our own pods, and whatever a group of octopi is, why not take a break, guy? To see the other whales for a bit." suggests Destiny

"Okay." says the others

So, Destiny, Hank, and Bailey swim off to do so, leaving Nemo, Marlin, Dory, Jenny, and Charlie alone.

"Why not go see our whale friend, not Destiny and Bailey, our Blue whale friend?" suggests Nemo

"That's a great idea." agrees Marlin; he's been working on his easy-going ways.

"Blue whale friend?" asks Jenny and Charlie

"Uh, huh! We made a whale friend before Marlin and Nemo meet you," says Dory

"Oh, how fun," says Jenny

"Yes. It is always good to make new friends," says Charlie

"Can we go introduce them to him, please, dad?" asked Nemo

"I don't see a problem in it," says Marlin

"Woohoo!" says Dory and Nemo

Marlin smiles, seeing them happy, so the gang goes and finds their friend.

"Mr. Whale, these are my parents Charlie and Jenny," says Dory

"Hello, Mr. Whale," says Charlie

"It's nice to meet you," says Jenny

The whale says it is a pleasure to meet them as well and asks if they want to play, which Dory translates.

"Yeah!" says Nemo, excited

"How do you play?" asks Charlie, confused

"We'll show you!" says Dory

Jenny and Charlie smile and follows the gang out in a distance where no one will bother them.

"He wants to know if we are ready to play." translates Dory

"Yup!" says Marlin and Nemo

"Uh.. sure," says Charlie and Jenny

The whale "swallows" the group, which confuses Jenny and Charlie.

"Mommy Daddy, just follow our lead," says Dory

"Alright dear," they say, trusting her

They all slide down the whale's tongue, and the whale sports them out of his hole on his head. They all laugh, enjoying that, and land on the bottom near the whale.

"So what did you think?" asks Nemo

"That was fun! Let's do that again!" says Jenny and Charlie

They smile and go again and again for a whole hour. The whale has a lot of fun with his fish friends, even his new fish friends. Soon it was time for the gang to meet up with Bailey, Destiny, and Hank again. So they told their whale friend goodbye and meet up with the trio.

"Did you guys have fun?" asks Bailey

"Oh yeah. Charlie and Jenny made a new friend," says Nemo

"That is wonderful," says Hank

"Yeah, we will come again," says Marlin

Daddy Son Day

A little while ago, before Nemo was ready to go to school, Marlin decides on a fun day just the two of them. He knows these moments are rare, and he needs to find the time with his son, especially after losing his wife at such a young Yesterday, Marlin let him play with the little kids but felt that he wasn't getting that bonding moment with Nemo. He was happy Nemo had a wonderful time but wanted to bond some more, so today, he is going to do something different.

"Where are we going, Daddy?" asks Nemo

"Oh, its a surprise," says Marlin

"Ooo a surprise?" says Nemo, happily

"Yeah," says Marlin

He holds Nemo's fin and leads him to a pirate ship.

"Okay, open," says Marlin

Nemo does, and he jumps about a little bit, getting excited.

"A pirate ship?!" exclaims Nemo

"Yup, we get to spend all day here just you and me," says Marlin

"Yay!" says Nemo, "Come on, daddy, I will race you."

"Alright! Ready set go!" says Marlin

Off the two go to the pirate ship, Marlin wins by an inch.

"Woo! " says Marlin

"Wow, you did amazing!" says Nemo

"Aw well, one day you will be just as good. You almost passed me," says Marlin

"I did?" asks Nemo

"Yeah, you did," says Marlin

Nemo beams at that, and so don't Marlin.

"Hey daddy can we go explore the pirate ship?" asks Nemo

"Of course. Maybe we will find a treasure chest," says Marlin

"That will be so cool!" says Nemo

"Yeah, it would be," says Marlin

The two swim off, looking at the pirate ship. They find the captain's quarters, where the crew slept, even some cannonballs and a small gaping hole.

"That looks like where a cannonball went through!" exclaims Nemo

He went closer to the hole.

"Careful Nemo, there might be sharp edges," warns Marlin

"I will. I just want to see it up close," says Nemo

He gets closer, marlin smiles, and lets him and looks closer at the cannon itself when he hears an ow.

"Gasp. Nemo!" says Marlin

He swims over to a crying Nemo.

"I saw something shiny hooked on the hole went to get it loose, and I slipped, and now my tummy hurts," says Nemo

"There there, let me see," says Marlin

Nemo lets Marlin see his tummy, there is a tiny scratch, but he can see why Nemo is in a lot of pain. He gives Nemo a cuddle and puts a little bit of seaweed on the wound, and holds Nemo close while he swims away from the pirate ship, comforting him the whole way.

"I think the shiny thing was meant to be there," says Marlin

"How come?" asks Nemo

"Well, because that is the shiny things home, and you wouldn't like it if someone tried to take you from your home, would you?" asks Marlin

"Nuh-uh. But it's so lonely, daddy," says Nemo

"I don't think it is lonely," says Marlin

"How come?" asks Nemo

"Well, because it has the pirate ship and the cannon and the seashells and the chest we never found to be its friend," says Marlin

"So he has many friends?" asks Nemo

"Yeah," says Marlin

"Yay. Will I have many friends?" asks Nemo

"Yeah, one day you will have lots and lots of friends," says Marlin

"Promise?" asks Nemo

"Promise," says Marlin

Nemo smiles then starts to think for a moment.

"I think the shiny should stay there then so he can make more friends," states Nemo

"That is a wonderful idea, Nemo. Come on, let's go home. When your better, we can go back and check to see if the shiny made new friends." says Marlin

"Okay," says Nemo

So they swim home, where Marlin takes care of the wound more and holds him close, humming a song that Coral taught him.

"I know that song," says Nemo

"Your mother use to sing it to you when you were in your egg," says Marlin

"Yeah. She had a beautiful voice," says Nemo

"Yeah, she did. She loved you a lot too," says Marlin

"She did?" asks Nemo

"Yeah, lots and lots," says Marlin

Nemo smiles then frowns.

"But she didn't know me," says Nemo

"That doesn't matter," says Marlin

Nemo looked up at him at that.

"It doesn't? But how can you love someone you don't know," asks Nemo

"Well, a mother loves their children unconditionally. There is a thing called unconditional love. That means that no matter what, even if they don't know you, they love you. Mothers and fathers have this kind of love with their children." says Marlin

"So even if the kid is bad, the mommy will love them?" asks Nemo

"Yes, even then. I promise now, and forever I will love you," says Marlin

Nemo smiles and hugs Marlin, which earns him a hug too.

"I will love you forever too," says Nemo

Marlin smiles and holds Nemo close, watching his stomach, knowing that even though for the moment Nemo forgot about the wound, the minute Marlin touches it, Nemo will remember and say ow. So, for now, he will let Nemo think that "daddies have the power to take the pain away."

Truth or Dare

Tonight the adults want to have a truth or dare game, so since Nemo is too young to know what that is, a lot of them are not appropriate for kids his age. Nemo is spending the night at Pearl's house with Tad and Sheldon. Tonight it is Dory, Hank, Bailey, Destiny, and Marlin; Marlin and Dory have been dating, so this makes it even more fun for the others. Hank is first, and Bailey has to ask him a question.

"Truth or Dare," asks Bailey

"Dare," says Hank, feeling adventurous

Bailey thought about that for a moment, trying to think of what to give Hank without boring him.

"I dare you to look like a human," says Bailey

"I haven't done that yet. Alright," says Hank

He concentrates and does so and quickly regrets it because humans can't breathe underwater. He quickly turns back.

"Okay! Let's not do that again!" quickly adds Destiny

"Agreed!" says everyone

"Okay, Bailey, truth or dare?" asks Destiny

Bailey thinks about this for a very long time, but the others come prepared, so end up playing the ocean version of go fish.

"I think I got it! I think I want to do uh...noooo...uh.." says Bailey

They sigh and continue playing for ten straight rounds of cards until they get annoyed with him.

"Just pick something! We all have to go to bed!" says everyone else

"Okay, Okay! Truth!" says Bailey

"Okay Bailey, if you went to school would you ditch on Senior Skip Day?" asks Destiny

"What?! No! I wouldn't miss out on a day of learning; also, that is terrifying! What happens if you get caught?!" asks Bailey

"Absolutely nothing," says Marlin

"You've done it before?" asks Bailey

"No, but other fish did and didn't get any repercussions," says Marlin

"Oh! Then...if I didn't do it alone, then maybe I would. Just maybe! It still sounds scary." says Bailey

"No, you wouldn't. We know you wouldn't unless we begged you too," says Dory and Destiny, knowing better.

Bailey blushes and smiles sheepishly.

"Ooo, it is your turn, Destiny, right? Truth or Dare," says Dory

"Dare!" says Destiny

"Yay! Okay, it is late, but erm...ooo! I don't want to forget this...Marlin! Where were we before the jellyfish?" asks Dory

"The trench?" ask Marlin

"Yeah, that place! I dare you to swim through it!" says Dory

Destiny gulped but nodded, so they decide to finish their game there and spend the night near there. They head over to it, watching where they were going as it was late. They finally make it there, and Destiny takes a deep breath. She heads in sideways and gasps when she makes out on the other side, okay.

"Guys, I did it!" she says excitedly

They all cheer happily and clap when she returns back to them; she bows happily.

"That was fun! Okay, Dory, your turn!" says Destiny

"Yay!" says Dory

"Okay, Dory, truth or dare," says Marlin

"Truth!" says Dory

"Okay...since we meet your parents, we know it doesn't run in your family, so how did you lose your memory?" asks Marlin

"Umm, I actually don't know I was told I was born with it," says Dory

"Ohhh," says everyone

"Okay Marlin, your turn," says Hank

"*gulp* Dare," says Marlin

He was worried because of Destiny's dare, but he wanted to try one too. Hank thought for a minute and whispers in Marlin's ear. Marlin turns red and grabs Dory's fin kissing her on the lips; she blinks but melts in the kiss. Marlin breaks it when they both need air.

"Wow..." says Dory

Marlin rubs the back of his head on that one.

"Aww," says the others

"Alright, I think it is time for bed," says Hank

They nod and go to bed away from where high traffic would be in the morning, falling asleep peacefully.

Dory Stays?

Dory smiled and watched as Marlin talked to Nemo. She is sad now because that means that she can't stay with them. She wants them to stay home but knows that she can't; she's just a friend of Marlin. He is a protective father, and she doubts that Marlin would let her stay with them.

"Dory! You helped my dad find me?" asks Nemo

"Huh? Oh, sorry, what was that, Elmo?" asks Dory

"Uh.Nemo. You helped my dad?" asks Nemo

"Oh yeah! I helped your dad, Nemo. It was a lot of fun too. Your such a great kid with a great dad." says Dory

"Yeah, I do. Oh! there are my friends!" says Nemo

"Go on, I am sure they missed you too," says Marlin

"Thanks, dad!" says Nemo; he swims over to where his friends are

"Um. I better go...I mean, we were only trying to save your son, right? Well ...now you have him. I better get back to what I was doing." says Dory

"Wait, at least let me help you home. I can see his friends right there. You shouldn't live too far from here." says Marlin. "Where do you live?"

"Um...I-I don't remember...I honestly don't think I ever had a home," says Dory

Marlin looks at her sad, knowing that is most likely true, or whatever home she had was probably taken. He doesn't know how long she has been swimming when they bumped into each other. The fact that she doesn't have a home is scary, but he doesn't know what to do.

"Let's swim and talk, okay? Tell me what you remember," says Marlin

"Okay, let's do that," says Dory

"Nemo! Stay there. I will be back in ten minutes!" says Marlin

"Okay, Dad!" says Nemo

Marlin swims with Dory; he was hoping she had a family to go home to know that they missed her. He would miss her because they bonded a lot these past few days. Who knows how long it has been since they started? He knows it has been a few days. Twenty four hours with one fish making friends, heck it has been him and Dory and Nemo on the way home. Nemo has been listening to the adventure here, so he hasn't really bonded with Dory. Though as far as Marlin can tell, they do like each other. Marlin listens as she tells him she was looking for something for days on days but can't remember what it was when she got distracted by a boat.

"Wait..so you don't have a home? You never had a home?" asks Marlin

"Not really, but I wasn't lonely; I meet a lot of nice fish," says Dory

"Really?" asks Marlin

"Yeah. It's okay," says Dory

"Dory, you need a place to call home," says Marlin

Marlin thinks for a minute and comes up with an idea.

"Hey Dory, can you do me a favour?" asks Marlin

"Sure!" says Dory

"I need to do something at my home, it's not that far, but I am worried about Nemo. He might remember how to get home, but he is a child. He shouldn't go home by himself," says Marlin

"Oh! I can take him home! He's the fish that looks like you, right?" asks Dory

"Exactly! Can you remember orange white strip fish?" asks Marlin

"Yeah!" says Dory

"Great! I will meet you both there. Stay with Nemo, and you will be on your way to my house," says Marlin

"Great!" says Dory

Marlin smiles and leaves, going home to make a surprise for Dory and Nemo, hoping that Nemo likes the idea. After a few minutes, Nemo comes over to Dory, all smiles he missed hanging out with them.

"Hey Dory, where is my dad?" asks Nemo

"Oh! He said he had to go home real quick and asked me to take you home. Do you know the way back from here?" asks Dory

"Yeah. Just follow me. We can talk on the way." says Nemo

"Great!" asks Dory, "Just to warn you, I suffer from short-term memory loss, so I'm sorry if we get lost."

"That's okay. I can find our way back," says Nemo

"Great!" says Dory

They start swimming some more, and they talk alot mainly on Nemo's side, as Dory listens to Nemo's side of the story getting excited.

"Wow, you are such a strong fish for someone so young! You are smart and brave too," says Dory

"You think?" asks Nemo, excited

"Oh yeah! If anyone can do all that at that age, that is very smart," says Dory

The connection grows as they swap stories and their likes and dislikes. Dory even teaches Nemo the "Just keep swimming" song. Marlin meets up with them and covers their faces.

"I have a surprise for you both!" says Marlin

"A surprise? I love surprises!" says Dory

"What surprise?" asks Nemo

"You'll see," says Marlin

He leads them to where Marlin and Nemo lives and uncovers their eyes where Marlin reveals that he dug a small hole and took a purple shell-like thing next to the sea anemone where Marlin and Nemo live.

"That is so cool! What is it ?" asks Dory and Nemo

"Well. Dory can't stay in the sea anemone because she will get shocked, so this is her new home," says Marlin

"Wait... Dory's staying?!" asks Nemo, sounding hopeful

"Well. If she wants to, is that alright?" asks Marlin

"Yeah! Please, Dory, please?" asks Nemo

"Are you serious?" asks Dory, smiling ear to ear

"Yeah. So what do you say? "asks Marlin

She hugs them both in response spinning them around.

"Is that a yes?" asks Nemo

"Yes!" says Dory

"Great, welcome home Dory and Nemo," says Marlin

"Welcome home."

The two smile and hug Marlin; Dory cuddles them both.

Dory is Teacher for A Day

Mr. Ray wasn't feeling too good and didn't want to cancel classes even though it would give the class a long weekend. He wasn't sure about this but had Dory take over for him. She was super excited and went over to his home.

"Dory? What are you doing here? Will the kids be expecting you soon? *cough* " asks Mr. Ray

"I know, but I wanted to ask you what I need to teach them today," says Dory, still excited

"Oh right, you know about sea turtles, right?" asks Mr. Ray

"Of course!" says Dory, remembering vaguely she spent two days with them.

"Great, I was going to save that for next week but go ahead and teach them about sea turtles," says Mr. Ray

"Great! I promise I will not let you down!" says Dory

She swims off and meets up with the kids.

"Where is Mr. Ray?" asks Kelly

"Well, he isn't feeling well today, and he doesn't want you guys to lose a day of learning, so I am your substitute teacher today!" says Dory

The kid's cheer; Dory was happy because she was nervous. They wouldn't like that.

"Okay! Today we will be learning about um..sea turtles! But first, don't you guys usually go somewhere?" asks Dory, taping her chin trying to remember

"The drop off" exclaims the kids

"Right the drop off! Follow me!" says Dory

She starts swimming but in the wrong direction.

"Other way!" says the kids

"Oh right, haha," says Dory

So they start going that way and get lost a few times but do manage to get there in less than an hour, which with Dory leading that is a miracle in itself, which the kids don't mind. They have fun with it.

"Okay, everyone gathers around," says Dory

A little green crab lifts his claw up.

"Ooo a question, yes?" asks Dory

"If Mr. Ray is called Mr. Ray because he is our teacher, what do we call you, Dory?" asks the green crab

"Oh right, teachers have titles, and I am a substitute teacher, right? Um...well anything you like, you can call me Dory or Miss Dory. Whatever you like is fine by me." says Dory

"Horray! " says the kids

"That was easy, um.., who knows a sea turtle?" asks Dory, all fins and claws shot up "wow, all of you?"

"Squirt was here for a bit." reminds Nemo

"Oh, right, here! Oh, better get started on teaching. Squirt and his father Crush live in the EAC. Does anyone know what the EAC stands for?" asks Dory

"East Australian Current?" asks a purple crab

"Correct! Sea turtles swim together in a bale. But they have other names um...*she thinks back* ooo! Nest and uh...turn and Dole." says Dory

"Ooooo," says the kids

"Can someone tell me what sea turtles eat?" asks Dory

"It depends on the type of sea turtle, achoo! Some turtles eat meat, some only eat plants, some eat both," says Sheldon

"Wow, you are really smart," said Dory

"Thanks," says Sheldon

"No problem here. Well, there is a lot to learn about sea turtles," says Dory

"Like what?" asks Pearl

"Well...ooh! Sea turtles can get up to 400 years old!" says Dory

"Wow!" says the kids

"What else?" asks Tad

"Um...oh! Sea turtles are found in warm and temperate waters," says Dory

Having lived in an aquarium, not that she remembers that, she knows a lot about sea and ocean creatures.

"Where did you learn that, Dory?" asks Nemo

"I am not sure actually, but I know its right; I think I read it somewhere," says Dory

The kids are confused by that but don't question it. They just enjoy the day learning about sea turtles and playing games. Near the end, they make Mr. Ray "get better soon" things until it's time to go home. The next week the kids surprise Mr. Ray with their creations.

"Wow! Thank you, kids; I love this. Did you guys have fun with Dory?" asks Mr. Ray

"Yes, Mr. Ray!" says the kids

"How would you feel about next time a sick she takes over again?" asks Mr. Ray

"Yay!" says the kids

"Great. What do we say to Dory?" asks Mr. Ray

"Thank you, Dory!" says the kids

"Aw. You guys. It was no problem; you guys were awesome. I had fun." says Dory

The kids smile, then it was time to learn something new for the day.

Dory Has A Sick Day

Nemo wakes up, Dory. You know she loves going with us to take you to school." says Marlin

"Okay!" says Nemo

He swims over to where Dory sleeps. Nemo pats her gently with his fin.

"Dory wake up, its time for me to go to school," says Nemo

"Oh school, I will be there soon," says Dory

Nemo nods and leaves, giving Dory room to move. Dory doesn't feel like moving because her stomach is hurting her. She feels awful; she knows deep down she shouldn't go to school, but she doesn't want to disappoint Nemo. She forces herself up and outside.

"I'm here. Let's go," says Dory

Marlin and Nemo look at her worried, Nemo couldn't really see in the darkness how bad she was. Marlin and Nemo swim over to her, worried.

"Dory, are you okay?" asks Nemo

They catch her before she gets lower.

"I am fine, just sleepy," says Dory, with a yawn

Marlin steadies her and brushes his fin on her forehead.

"Dory, you're burning up!" says Marlin, "Nemo, help me get her back to bed."

"No, no, Nemo has to go to school," says Dory

"It's okay, Dory your sick; you need to rest." says Nemo, "You can take me when you're better."

Marlin and Nemo get her into her home to rest.

"Are you sure?" asks Dory

"Yes. Rest okay?" asks Nemo

"Alright," says Dory

It wasn't long for Dory to fall back asleep; Merlin and Nemo look at her sadly and start heading toward Nemo's school.

"Will she be okay, Dad?" asks Nemo

"She will be fine. Come on, your going to be late," says Marlin

They swim there and make it to where Mr. Ray was waiting for Nemo.

"There you are! Is Dory not joining us today?" asks Mr. Ray

"No, she isn't feeling well today," says Nemo

Mr. Ray looks at Marlin for guidance.

"She is showing signs of a stomach ache," says Marlin

"Well, I am sorry to hear that. I hope she feels better. But for now, Nemo lets learn for her, okay?" asks Mr. Ray

"Okay," says Nemo; he swims up Mr. Ray

"I really do hope that Dory feels better," says Mr. Ray

"Thank you. I better get back to her before she forgets that I sent him to school," says Marlin

Mr. Ray nods and lets Marlin go, which Marlin is glad he made it back home to stop Dory from leaving the bed.

"Dory, back to bed; you're sick," says Marlin

"Nemo is late for school, though," says Dory

"He was almost late; I got him there on time," says Marlin

"Oh, why wasn't I woke up?" asks Dory

"You were, but you weren't feeling well, so we asked you to stay in bed," says Marlin

"You did?" asks Dory

"Yes, please rest, okay? You look like your stomach is hurting you," says Marlin

She goes to act like she's fine, but she has another pain in her stomach and nods. Marlin helps her back into bed and takes care of the rest of the day; she sleeps most of the day. Marlin doesn't mind; he lets her sleep and gets Nemo. He has him keep quiet, so Dory can rest the rest of the day. Nemo agrees happily to do so.

"Can I help take care of Dory, dad?" asks Nemo

"Sure, Nemo. I am sure she will like that," says Marlin, with a smile.

Nemo smiles and helps Marlin with Dory; it takes a few days for Dory to feel better. But when she does, she is even bubblier than ever. She hugs Nemo and Marlin.

"Thank you for taking care of me," says Dory

They smile and hug her back happily.

"It was not a problem, Dory," they say

They enjoy the rest of the day at the park with Dory jumping around, making Nemo and Marlin very happy.

Hiccup Tricks

Marlin is trying to show Dory some adult fun. He knows that sometimes talking to adults isn't all that fun sometimes, but Dory is an adult and should be treated as such. He noticed that she really loves jokes. So he starts telling her some jokes, making her laugh.

"Oh, I have another one ready for it?" asks Marlin, smiling

"Okay," says Dory, laughing

He starts telling her about the sea mollusc joke that he messed up a few times, but now he remembers it, so he tells her— making her laugh harder and harder until she has hiccups.

"Dory, careful you're getting hiccups," says Marlin

"It's okay *hiccup* they will go away soon. *hiccup* I have gotten them before, at least I think I did," says Dory hiccuping again

"Alright," says Marlin

So they swim on, and Marlin shows her how chores could be fun, and they end up dancing while Dory hiccups the whole time.

"Uh oh, they aren't going away," says Dory

She isn't all that worried about that, but she finds it weird.

"Let's try some tricks to get rid of them," says Marlin

"Okay! " says Dory

"Try holding your breath for a minute. I will do it with you," says Marlin

She nods and follows his lead holding her breath. They hold it for a whole sixty seconds and then let out a long breath.

"Did it work?" asks Marlin

She starts hiccuping again for a long time this time.

"That would be no," says Marlin

"Well, let's not give up *hiccup* Let's try something else," says Dory

"Okay, oh, wait there," says Marlin

"Alright," says Dory

He swims away and hides, knowing she will get bored and start looking. This is exactly what happens, and when she swims past him while she is hiccuping, he jumps up and yells, boo scaring her.

"Ahhh!" says Dory, "Why did you do that? *hiccup*."

"Well, I was trying to scare your hiccups away," says Marlin

"Ooo did it *hiccup*, work?" asks Dory

"No.," says Marlin

"Aw *hiccup*, "says Dory

"It's okay; I have a couple more tricks," says Marlin

"Alright. Like what?" asks Dory

"Oh well, the first one is covering your mouth for a few minutes," says Marlin

So they try that swimming with their tail around heading back, Nemo was left with Jenny and Charlie, and they are both sure he is ready to go home by now. It works for a little bit but then Dory hiccups again.

"This one is a little more fun," says Marlin

"Ooo fun, what exactly?" asks Dory

"Well, you flip upside down and swim backward while holding your breath," says Marlin

"That does sound like fun! Let's do it!" says Dory

Marlin smiles and joins her, all the way to Jenny and Charlie's where they meet up with Nemo. Nemo sees this and laughs, watching his father and Dory swim upside down. They flip over before they get a headache.

"Hi Nemo!" says Dory, "Ooo, no hiccups! It worked! Haha!"

"Is that why you were upside down dear?" asks Jenny

"Marlin was helping me with my hiccups," says Dory

Marlin rubs his head sheepishly.

"Isn't that so?" asks Charlie, with a smile

"Well, I knew a few tricks, so tried to help after they didn't go away after a few minutes," says Marlin

"Well, whatever you two did worked," says Charlie

"Yeah, I haven't heard Dory hiccup since you two came up here," says Nemo

"Really? Yay!" says Dory

They smile at that happily, and after thanking Charlie and jenny for babysitting, they start home, where Nemo tells Dory and Marlin about their day.

Harmony

One day Dory was exploring, and she finds a baby fish; she is a teal and green fish.

"Aww. What's your name?" asks Dory

"Harmony," says the baby fish

"Where're your parents?" asks Dory

"I dunno," says Harmony, her eyes watering

"Don't cry. Don't worry. I have friends, and we can figure this all out." says Dory

"Really?" asks Harmony

"Of course," says Dory

She takes Harmony home with her and explains the situation. Nemo and Marlin agree to help her by looking for the baby's parents for her. Dory sits down and plays with the baby fish until it gets late. After dinner, she holds the baby fish close and can't think of any stories to tell the baby fish but does think of songs she could sing to the baby. She rocks Harmony and thinks for a minute.

"Dory?" asks Harmony

"Just thinking," says Dory

"Okay," says Harmony

"Lullaby, and goodnight, in the skies stars, are the moon's silvery beams bring you sweet your eyes now and rest, may these hours be blessed.'Til the sky's bright with dawn, when you wake with a, and goodnight, you are mother's delight.

I'll protect you from harm, and you'll wake in my, close your eyes, for I'm right beside angels are near, so sleep without, and good night, with roses o'er head, lay thee down in thy, and goodnight, you are mother's delight. I'll protect you from harm, and you'll wake in my, and sleep tight, my darling sheets white as cream, with a head full of, close your eyes, I'm right beside thee down now and rest, may your slumber be blessed.

Go to sleep, little one, think of puppies and to sleep, little one, think of butterflies into sleep, little one, think of bright sunny morning', darling one, sleep through the night, Sleep through the night, Sleep through the night." sings Dory

Harmony yawns and falls asleep easily. Dory smiles and falls asleep. The next day starts playing with Harmony, and Harmony giggles and ends up getting hiccups, which cause Dory to get a hiccup.

"Uh *hiccup* oh," says Harmony

"It will *hiccup* be okay. *hiccup*" says Dory

Dory helps Harmony with the hiccups and stops the hiccups. It takes a while, but they get it done. Harmony is still full of energy, so Dory and Nemo play some games with her until Nemo has to go to bed. Then Dory plays with her all night with Harmony until the next morning she is asleep. Dory is tired, but she can't do anything about it. She has to eat and make sure that everything else is going okay. Today her parents are staying with

Jenny and Charlie while Dory, Nemo, and Marlin go out looking with that lead. They spend the whole day waiting at the house of the possible parents but nothing.

"We will come tomorrow, dory. You look exhausted. You should go home," says Marlin

"*yawn* Alight," says Dory

She heads home and settles down for a nap. When she wakes up, Harmony is whiny in the makeshift crib; Dory scoops her up and holds her close.

"Shh, Shh. *starts rocking Harmony* Hush, little baby, don't say a word, Mama's going to buy you an if that mockingbird doesn't sing, Mama's going to buy you a diamond ring.

And if that diamond ring turns brass, Mama's going to buy you a looking if that looking glass gets broke, Mama's going to buy you a billy if that billy goat doesn't pull,

Mama's going to buy you a cart, and if that cart and bull turn over, Mama's going to buy you a dog named if that dog named Rover won't bark, Mama's going to buy you a horse, and if that horse and cart fall down, You'll still be the sweetest little baby in town." sings Dory

Harmony falls asleep again; Dory sighs and puts her back to bed, and goes back to bed herself. The next morning Nemo and Marlin go off back to the leads house.

"Dory?" asks Harmony

"Yes?" asks Dory

"Does this mean they found Mama and Daddy?" asks Harmony

"Possibly," says Dory

"Can you sing me a song before they come to pick me up?" asks Harmony

"Sure," says Dory

She starts to sing Rock abye baby, but Harmony stops her.

"Noo. Not a lullaby. Something that has a lullaby in it." says Harmony

"Oh hmm," says Dory

She thinks about it for a minute and remembers Rockabye by Clean Bandit. (if you want to listen to the song over-reading all this, I understand)

"Call it love, and it the mom's adoration, foundation. A special bond of creation, hah For all the single mums out through Bandit, Sean-Da-Paul, Anne-marie, sing, make them works the night, by the 's gonna stress, so far away from her father's just wants a life for her on her own, no one will 's got to save tells him "ooh love."No one's ever gonna hurt you, love. I'm gonna give you all of my love. Nobody matters like tells him, "your life ain't gonna be nothing like my life. You're gonna grow and have a good life. I'm gonna do what I've got to do" So, Rockabye baby, Rockabye, I'm gonna rock baby, don't you 's got baby, Rockabye. I'm gonna rock baby, don't you cry. Rockabye, yeah, yeah. Mom, what are you doing out there?

Facing a hard life without fear. Just see and know that you really care.'Cause any obstacle to come you well prepared And no mamma you never shed a tear.'Cause you have set things year after you give the youth love beyond finding the school fee and the bus more when paps a wrong bar can't find him anywhere. Steadily you workflow, heavily you know so you nah stop. No time fi she gotta six-year-old. Trying to keep him to keep all the looks her in the don't know he's safe when she says."Ooh, love, "No one's ever gonna hurt you, love. I'm gonna give you all of my matters like Rockabye baby, Rockabye. I'm gonna rock baby, don't you 's got baby, Rockabye. I'm gonna rock baby, don't you, yeah. don't bother up your head, lift it up to the sky, don't bother around you, just joy your she gotta six-year to keep him to keep all the looks her in the doesn't know he's safe when she says." sings Dory

Marlin and Nemo return with the parents, but the parents stop Marlin and Nemo from interrupting Dory from singing to their daughter.

"She tells him, "ooh love, "No one's ever gonna hurt you, love. I'm gonna give you all of my matters like tells him, "your life ain't gonna be nothing like my life. You're gonna grow and have a good life. I'm gonna do what I've got to do".So, Rockabye baby, Rockabye. I'm gonna rock baby, don't you 's got you Rockabye baby, Rockabye. I'm gonna rock baby, don't you? Rockabye, don't bother up your head, lift it up to the sky, yo Rockabye! Rockabye, don't bother around you; just joy your eye, Rockabye! Rockabye, don't bother up your head, lift it up to the sky, yo Rockabye! Rockabye don't bother to cry Angels around you, just joy your eye." sings Dory

The parents go over, and Harmony hugs them, and Dory smiles happily to see them together.

"Thank you." says the parents

"Aw, it's nothing. I'm just glad she can be safe at home again," says Dory

The parents smile. Happily, Harmony swims and hugs Dory; Dory hugs back before they leave.

Hide and Go Find Dory

Destiny, Hank, and Bailey came over to hang out with Dory, Nemo, and Marlin today. They were starting to get bored after a long morning of talking and catching up. Destiny and Bailey made more whale friends while Hank, on the other hand, was more of a loner and just hung out with a few acquaintances. The three bumped into each other yesterday, and Hank stayed with the duo then next morning decided to visit Marlin, Dory, and Nemo.

"So uh...what do we do now?" asks Hank

"Ooo, how about hiding and go seek!" suggests Dory

"Yeah!" says the others

So they play a few rounds taking turns of playing the person who would seek. Dory wasn't having any luck when it was her turn to hide because she would forget what they were doing and would reveal herself or pick the same hiding spot. This was rare with Dory, as she was usually good at hiding and went seeking. It was getting dark soon, so this would be the last turn.

"Psst dory come here." whispers Destiny

Dory smiles and comes over to where Destiny was hiding while Hank counted.

"How about we work together," suggests Destiny

"Okay. How?" asks Dory

"I hide, and you hide in my mouth." says Destiny, "then I pretend that I don't know where you are," says Destiny

"You okay. I like it," says Dory

So she swims into Destiny's mouth and hides behind Destiny's tonsils so Destiny could talk, and Dory wouldn't be found. The game continued, and this time, Nemo was found first, and Destiny was found last, not including Dory. So the gang teamed up and continued looking for Dory. Destiny knew she would have to give up Dory's hiding spot soon, but right now, she was having too much fun. However, the further they went, the harder it became for Destiny to tell them. A couple of hours pass by, and Destiny forgets herself where Dory was hiding.

"Dory!" they all call

They gather where the original spot where they started out and asked everyone where they looked for her.

"Did you find her?" asks Hank

"No," says Nemo

"Not a sign of her," says Marlin

"We looked everywhere," says Bailey

"Yeah, we couldn't find her," says Destiny

Dory was confused about why Destiny didn't tell them where she was.

"Hey!" calls Dory

Everyone froze and looked around, confused themselves.

"Can I come out now?!" asks Dory

"Yes! You win!" they all say

"Yay! Uh, Destiny, can you open up?" asks Dory

"Oh, that's right! Silly me!" says Destiny

She opened up and let Dory out.

"We make a great team!" says Dory

"Yeah, we do!" says Destiny

They high five the others blinked but smiled at the two.

"You two did great jobs, kids," says Hank

The two smile at that, and then it was time to eat; it was too late for Hank, Bailey, and Destiny to go home, so they all had a sleepover. It was a wonderful night.

Baby Boy

Marlin took the egg and cooked the egg with him to bed with him too afraid to leave the egg in the hole he and Coral dug alone. He cuddles with his baby and fell asleep. The next morning it really sunk in what happened, and he couldn't help but cry. He felt something rolling around and got up.

"Oh! Sorry Nemo, daddy is going to be okay. I am right here, baby boy. I promise." says Marlin.

He scooped up his egg and cuddled it. He carried the egg around all day, ignoring the whispers and looks.

"Ignore them, Nemo; they don't know what they are talking about. This is going to be your town one day," says Marlin

He swam on with his egg and protected his baby from all ends of the ocean. He even shows the egg where Nemo would be playing before school.

"Hey mister, why are you carrying an egg around?" asks a little boy

"He's going to be my baby soon," says Marlin

"Joel! Be nice. I am so sorry," says Joel's mom

"No, it is okay; he is just asking a question, I don't mind," says Marlin

The mom nods with a shy smile.

"Oh, wow! Is the baby a boy or a girl?" asks Joel

"I won't know until the baby is born. But if the baby is a boy, his name is going to be Nemo," says Marlin

"Nemo? That is a cool name! Um. if your his daddy, then where is his mommy?" asks Joel

"Joel!" warns his mom

"It's okay; he is a kid he doesn't know. *to Joel* Well, there was an accident, and his mommy is gone now; she was killed yesterday," says Marlin

"Oh..." says Joel,

"I am so sorry," says Joel's mom

Marlin can only nod; Joel grabs a flower and lays it on top of the egg.

"Mommy says flowers help people when they are sad. That is for Nemo and you," says Joel

Marlin smiles and gives Joel a pat on the head.

"Thank you, Joel. I have to go home now, but I am sure that when Nemo is born, he will love this flower," says Marlin

Joel beams and lets Marlin goes off. Marlin has to eat so he can be there for Nemo when he is born; Marlin eats, keeping an eye on Nemo's egg. He plays with the flower after putting the egg to bed. He smiles and falls asleep; the next day, he takes the egg out, and Joel found them.

"It's Nemo and his daddy! Hi Nemo!" says Joel

"Hi there, Joel," says Marlin

"Can I talk to Nemo for a bit?" asks Joel

"Uh sure," says Marlin

He lets Joel talk to Nemo and even hold the egg reluctantly. Marlin even talks to Joel's mom before it was time for Joel to go home. Marlin smiles, wishing Joel was younger so that Nemo could get to know him better. He knows once it's time for Nemo to go to school, Joel will already be a teenager and might not remember Nemo. He swims off and relaxes with Nemo. For the next few weeks, he never left Nemo's side, and a couple of times, he ran into Joel again; they ended up being friends. The flower was starting to wilt, so Joel got him a new flower so Nemo can enjoy the beauty too. One morning Marlin felt movement in the egg. He woke up and gasped when he saw the egg hatch. He hugged his baby close. After the excitement, he checked to see if the baby is a boy or a girl.

"Hi Nemo, I am your daddy, and look, your friend Joel gave you this," says Marlin

He shows Nemo the flower, Nemo smiles at the flower happily.

Crystal Shell

Dory and her friends were playing out in the open ocean far out of the town. They have never been anywhere near there before, so it was very interesting to them. Dory sees something gleaming at the bottom of the ocean, so she goes and gets it. It turns out to be a crystal shell; she shows her friends.

"Guys! Look what I found!" says Dory

"What is it?" asked Nemo

They all swam over to find out what she found.

"It looks like a crystal shell," says Marlin

"Ooh," says the others

"Aw, that sounds important. I better keep hold of it just in case someone comes looking for it," says Dory

"Are you sure, Dory?" asks Marlin. "That is a huge responsibility."

"Oh yeah. It is so pretty and lonely looking," says Dory

"Sigh. Alright. You can keep it." says Marlin

"Yay! Come on guys, let's go find a special place for this shell at my place.!" says Dory

Little did they know a guard fish saw this and swam after they worried something bad would happen to it. Little did he know that this trip took them three days to get home, but lucky for him, he made it to the group in time as they were camping out little ways out, close as they could get from their home. They left right after Nemo got out of school, so they couldn't stay for more than a couple of hours, so Nemo would miss one day of school over two.

"Halt!" says the guard

The gang does and jumps at his sudden appearance; Nemo is held close by his father.

"Who are you?" asks Hank

"I am a royal guard to a sea princess." says the guard; he shows them proof making them gasp.

"That shell you have is very important to my princess."

"If it is so important, why doesn't she have it now?" asks Marlin, in a non-mean way

"An evil sea witch took it from her. She hid it in the sand before she was captured, but we had no clue where. I was the one looking around this area on my shift. I must bring it back to her." says the guard

"What will happen if you don't?" asks Bailey

"The princess has become weak without the power, and without it, she will die." says the guard

The crew gasps, and Dory goes to gently hand it back, but it shocks him.

"It seems the shell doesn't want to go home with me. I must ask you a favor, young one." says the guard

"Uh.. okay," says Dory

"Will you come back to me to the palace and deliver this to the princess?" asks the guard

"Can my friends come?" asks Dory

"Of course. But may I ask your names?" asks the guard

So everyone introduced themselves, and the guard took note of this.

"Very well, we must not take to long; it is already a two-day trip back to the palace." says the guard

They nod and then swim back to the palace began; they were making good time as well, especially with the guard protecting them and the crystal shell. However, on the second day, as the princess was lying on her deathbed, so was the crystal shell.

"We must hurry!" says the guard

That night they all went without sleep and headed further to the castle. Which the guard had to tell the main guard what happened before they were allowed in. But because of how ill the princess was, only Dory was allowed to see her, which the others didn't mind. So Dory followed the guard to the princess's room.

"Hi your majesty, I have something for you," says Dory

The princess looked at her, even as week as she was anyone could tell she is very beautiful. Dory gives the shell to the princess, suddenly there was a power boost, and both the princess and the shell were looking so much better.

"Thank you." says the Princess, "I am forever in your debt. I can't talk right now, but if you could leave your address, I will come to see you when I am well."

"Aw, it is okay; you just get some rest," says Dory

She smiles and comes out where everyone was waiting on the edge of their fins.

"She's going to make it," says Dory

Everyone in the palace cheered loudly.

"Wait for guys, she's resting," says Dory

They cover their mouths and cheer quieter, Dory explains what happened, and Marlin leaves the address with the guard.

"For helping our daughter, we would love to give you a ride home." says the king

"Oh, thank you!" says everyone

So in the carriage, they go, and they ride to Nemo's school in style where Nemo gets dropped off, and everyone else goes home.

"Thank you for the ride," says Marlin

"Not a problem. You all are now welcome guests anytime." says the king

"Always," says the queen

Dory and Marlin's smile watching the King and Queen, left happily.

Bedtime

It is late at night, and Nemo wakes up. He can't sleep; he doesn't want to wake his dad up and knows that Dory stays up sometimes. So he swims over to where Dory is just falling asleep.

"Dory," says Nemo

"Huh? Nemo, why are you up?" asks Dory

"I can't sleep.," states Nemo

"Aw well, come snuggle in here with me, and I will tell you a story," says Dory

Nemo smiles and curls up next to Dory.

"All comfy?" asks Dory

"Uh-huh," says Nemo

"Great um.." starts Dory; she tries to think of a non-girly story and remembers that he loves pirates. "Ooo, I know!...

Dory starts out the story:

Once upon a time, there was the best pirate in the world; his name was Blackbeard. Blackbeard had a pirate crew so tough that no one wanted to stand in his way. He could have all the ships he wanted and all the gold and jewels he wanted. He loved sailing the seas and finding new things and new lands. His heart belonged to the waters, however. His ship's name was uh...Queen Anne's Revenge"

"Wow, he worked for a queen?!" asks Nemo in awe

"Uh-huh," says Dory

"Did he have a love life?" wonders Nemo; like most children his age, he was wondering about the love life

She continues the story:

Oh yeah, her name was Mary Ormond; Blackbeard would do anything for her. He carried around her scarf on his pirate hat. No one ever made fun of him because they knew if they had a woman like Mary, they would do the same thing. She was the smartest and most loyal woman he ever laid eyes on, very beautiful as well. His heart was hers, but she knew she could never take him from the sea. So off, Blackbeard went on another adventure where he stayed out for months out looking for more treasures and land.

"I bet he was looking for the best for Mary," states Nemo, with a yawn

"Oh yeah, only the best for Mary and his crew," says Dory

She continues:

However, when he got what he wanted, a newcomer came to attack his ship and take all his hard-earned jewels. His name was um...Jewelry Bonney. He had his ship get up to where Blackbeard's ship was, and after the cannons were being shot, Jewelry went over to where Blackbeard was, and the two started fighting like men with their swords and fists. The battle continued on for a few minutes.

'Give up, old man!' says Jewelry

'Never! Just get out of the way and start home !' states Blackbeard

Jewelry trips Blackbeard, but Blackbeard found Jewelry's weakness in his knee. So Blackbeard took the backend of his sword and bashed Jewelry's knee, making Jewelry back off in pain. Blackbeard put the same sword to Jewelry's throat.

'I will tell you once call your crew to retreat or die.' says Blackbeard

Jewelry wasn't willing to die yet, so he did as told and left with his life. Blackbeard checked on everything else and then continued on his way home. "

Dory finishes and sees Nemo fast asleep. She smiles and follows his lead falling asleep. The next morning Marlin wakes up and panics, seeing Nemo is gone. He swims out and freezes, seeing Dory and Nemo fast asleep. Marlin smiles and relaxes, deciding to let them sleep in.

Sleeping With Gil

Dory and Marlin stop their search for food, knowing that searching while hungry won't make anything better. In the meantime, Nemo just finished and failed to try to get rocks in the machine. He felt awful about it; Gil looks at him feeling awful about it.

"Gil. Talk to him," says Peach

"What do I say? I never dealt with a kid before," says Gil

"Anything but is gentle. He might feel like he failed you. He misses his dad." says Peach

"Yeah, I know; I will talk to him," says Gil

"Good," says Peach

Gil swam up to Nemo as he was taking a deep breath.

"Hey, Shark bait," says Gil

Nemo jumps and sees Gil.

"Oh...hey Gil. Gil? I am sorry. I messed everything up." says Nemo

"Nah. Don't worry about it. It happens. How many times do you think I failed?" asks Gil

"Uh...I am not sure," says Nemo

"Over one hundred times," says Gil

"Really?" asks Nemo

"Yeah, really. It happens, kiddo. Trust me, if I didn't fail wed all be out here, and you would be stuck here still with other fish." says Gil

"Wow. You have a good point. Gil? Will we be able to get out of here one day?" asks Nemo

"I am sure of it. One day you will get back with your dad. And we all will be free." says Gil

Nemo smiles at that happily.

"Enough of that talk, come on, let's get something to eat. I want to tell you some stories," says Gil

"Okay," says Nemo

So they grabbed something to eat, and Gil tells him how the others got here, all of course from pet stores as they said. Gil the only one from the ocean, just like Nemo.

"I would tell them stories of the ocean; some scared them, but more than anything, they wanted to go to the ocean, just like I wanted to go back. However, every attempt, we always ended up back in here," says Gil

"How did you end up here?" asks Nemo

"Me? I was zapped by jellyfish when I was little. I went swimming and got caught on the rocks. The dentist captured me, took care of my wound, and I have been here ever since." says Gil

"...wow," says Nemo

"Yeah. How about you, Nemo?" says Gil

"...nothing like that. " starts Nemo

Nemo says his story and listens to Nemo's whole story.

"I see. So you and your old man had a fight, and you ended up kidnapped after touching the boat," says Gil

"Y-yeah," says Nemo

"I bet your dad is looking for you right now," says Gil

"For me? After everything," asks Nemo

"If I was your dad, yeah. Mine probably thinks I am dead. But you? You have been gone for a few days. I am sure he is looking now. He loves you a lot." says Gil

Nemo smiles and looks out the window again.

"Yeah," says Nemo

"Come on, its time for bed," says Gil

"Alright, Gil," says Nemo

So they all went to bed after that. However, Gil's words of "if we escaped, different fish would be here right now" haunted him more than he thought, and he has a nightmare.

In Nightmare:

Nemo wakes from a nightmare and sees other fish. He flies around and goes to one that looks like bubbles.

"Hey bubbles, why aren't you near your chest watching your chest?" asks Nemo

"Go away. I don't have time for your dumb questions, Nemo. And why would I be near a dumb chest?" asks Bubbles, "and the name ain't bubbles! I told you that before."

"Uh...I was told your name was bubbles. Sorry." says Nemo

He goes up to Deb.

"Auntie Deb? Is something wrong with bubbles?" asks Nemo

"Deb? Am I Flo whos deb? And whos bubbles. Did you bother old-growth again? We told you to stay away from him." says Flo

"Uh...okay..." says Nemo

He swims over to Jaques, he doesn't know French, but Jaques does understand English.

"Jaques? Everyone is acting weird you know what is going on?" asks Nemo

Jaques keeps on swimming, not knowing what he said.

"Jaques?" says Nemo

"He doesn't understand English. How many times must you be told?" asks Gurgle

"What are you talking about? He understood when you asked for me to get clean.

"Why would I care if your clean or not?" asks Gurgle

"You always have," says Nemo

"No, I haven't," says Gurgle

"Kid, you okay? You know he likes things messy," says Bloat

"No, that's you," says Nemo

"No, I like it clean," says Bloat

Nemo gets worried and goes to Peach.

"Sweetie, you okay?" asks Peach

"N-no. Everything is weird, Peach," says Nemo

"Well, you know what else is weird you calling me Peach and being near me? Go away! When are you even here instead of that skull of yours?" asks Peach

"What are you talking about? That is where Gil lives," says Nemo

"Whos girl? There is no girl here," says Peach

Nemo panics and goes looking for Gil but can't find him. When he looks in a picture, he sees Darla holding a bag with Gil upside down. He gasps and burst awake. He swims to Gil's skull and curls up next to him, breathing hard.

"Shark bait?" asks Gil

"S-sorry...just a nightmare," says Nemo

Gil looks at his scared fast and relaxes.

"It is alright, Nemo. You can sleep here tonight," says Gil

"You sure?" asks Nemo

"Yeah," says Gil

"Thanks, Gil," says Nemo, smiling.

"No problem," says Gil

They fall back asleep, Nemo, with a smile on his face.

Alternative Fish

There are seven lookalikes in the world; this doesn't count out animals either; Dory finds that out quick one day while swimming around the Great Barrier Reef, she ends up daydreaming and bumps into an outside fish.

"Watch where you're going!" says the female fish

"Ouch. So sorry. *she looks at the fish* You look familiar," says Dory

"Is it while looking in a mirror because I look like you? Now move." says the female fish

"Oh, you do! Hi twin, I think that's the term; I'm Dory," says Dory

"Twin?" asks the female fish

"Uh, huh. That's what fish is that look the same. But I don't believe I have a twin sister. You look like me, though." says Dory
The fish looked at her strangely but nods.

"Magnolia. Don't ever call me that," says Magnolia

"What do you want to be called?" asks Dory

"Call me Mags," says Mags

"Okay, Mags. Oh! Are you busy?" asks Dory

"A bit, I have to find a new place to crash for the night and secure it as mine," says Mags

"Oh..ooo! Why not come stay with me?" asks Dory

"Because we just meet weirdo," says Mags

"I know that silly, but it's better than going place to place and being alone, isn't it?" asks Dory

Mags thought about it for a minute and looked at Dory; it was clear who the more dangerous one is. She shrugs and smiles at Dory.

"Alright, Dory. Lead the way to your place," says Mags

Dory smiles at that and leads Mags to where Marlin and Nemo are waiting for her.

"Guys! Look! It's my twin!" says Dory

"Sup," says Mags

"Uh..hi..." says Marlin and Nemo

"Her name is Mags. She's going to be staying with me for a while until she can find somewhere else to stay," says Dory

"What she said," says Mags

"Uh, what? Dory, can I talk to you for a minute?" asks Marlin

"Sure!" says Dory

They go over to talk about it.

"Want to play a game?" asks Nemo

"Sure, kid," says Mags

They play together in plain sight, so Marlin doesn't flip out

"She can't stay here! We don't know a thing about her!" says Marlin

"I know that, Marlin, but she was alone and had nowhere to go," says Dory

"What do you mean?" asks Marlin

"I mean, she was looking for a place to crash when I meet her. What was I supposed to do, let her stay in the cold? She seems really nice, and Nemo likes her." says Dory

She points to Nemo and Mags playing fish tag. Marlin thinks about what she just said and looked at Nemo, having fun.

"Okay. Okay, she can stay," says Marlin

"Great! Thanks!" says Dory

They go over to her and get her situated with Dory. Mags meets all their friends over the next few weeks and even sees everything they own, including a shiny crown.

"($.$) Hello!" says Mags

"Mags? Aren't you going to the store with me?" asks Jenny

"Oh yeah, might even look at homes while I'm at it," says Mags

"Okay dear," says Jenny

"Hey, Jen. Where did this crown come from?" asks Mags.

"Oh, that. It's a gift from a friend of ours. Don't worry about it, honey. Come along." says Jenny

Mags looks at the crown and leaves with Jenny. There has been a lot of theft going around the Great Barrier reef, but no one knows why. Of course, everyone blames Mags, but Dory defends her the whole time. Mags takes very bad advantage of that; she has a huge debt to go over with a mafia fish, so she steals what she can only give a small chunk to the mafia; they are the reason she is homeless, to begin with. Actually, it is her fault because she stole from them once and sold it to another look-alike, who ended up in trouble because of that, but she ended up with the debt over her look-alike because that look alike couldn't see that well. That night, she decides to take the crown, and as there is a campout outside of Jenny and Charlie's house, then this works out well. She swims inside once everyone is asleep and sees the crown.

"Bingo, hi gorgeous, you are going to get me out of so much trouble," says Mags

"Mags? What are you doing?" asks Dory

Mags quickly hides the crown and looks at Dory.

"I was uh..just taking a walk," says Mags

She knows that Dory is dumb, but Dory notices that the fin is bent back; she moves the fin and sees the crown.

"You were going to steal after my parents?! After everything.." says Dory

She takes the crown back, and looks at it, then starts putting two and two together; there were times that Mags would disappear for several minutes.

"Where is everything else?" asks Dory

"Huh?" says Mags

"Where. Is. Everything. Else?! You stole from everyone! Where is it?!" asks Dory

"Gone," says Mags. "And guess what, sugar, this isn't a thing you can do about it."

Dory glares at that, grab her fin rough and drag her with her.

"Get off! Dory, hey!" says Mags

Dory ignores her, gripping harder; she leads her to the sunken ship where Chum, Bruce, and Anchor live.

"Are you crazy?! Don't you know there are sharks here?!" asks Mags, fighting against Dory's grip

"Yup," says Dory

"Yet you're taking us to our death?!" asks Mags

She is really frightened right now, which anyone would be going to see sharks. Dory ignores her and brings her inside.

"Dory!" says the happy sharks

"It's been forever!" says Anchor

"Yeah! You need to come to see us more. Who's your friend?" asks Chum

"Oh, believe me, she is no friend of mine," says Dory

The three look at her then at each other.

"Dory, what's wrong?" asks Bruce

Dory explains everything and that she caught Mags red-handed.

"And she won't tell me where anything is!" says Dory

"Oh, she won't now? Well, maybe we can help with that, Shelia," says Bruce

"Thanks, guys. She's all yours," says Dory

She lets go and lets the boys handle her.

"I'll talk, I'll talk!" says Mags

"Then get talking," says Chum

"I know where the stuff is, but I wasn't stealing them for myself. I was stealing them because I owe money. A lot of money. The fish who I owe is the reason I have no home, and he won't let me go or give me back my home until I give them the money back. They got back what I stole back, but that wasn't enough for them. I owe them for what it is the cost!" says Mags

"So you're a thief who stole from the wrong person," says Chum

"Basically. Look, I am just trying to pay for my debt and get my house back," says Mags

They all talk about it for a moment, then come back.

"We will help you out of your mess and get your house back on one condition," says Bruce

"Of course, there is a condition. What?" asks Mags

"You personally return the stuff you stole, and then you quit your theft ways," says Bruce

"Or what?" asks Mags

"Or we will kick you out for good; no one will let you anywhere near the other towns," says Anchor

"Like sharks, no one wants to mess with us," says Chum

"Okay! Okay, fine," says Mags

So the five of them go talk to the person she stole from and got the goods and her house back. They then make her go door to door to give the stuff back with an explanation. Then they leave her in her house.

"Thanks, guys," says Dory

"Not a problem, anything for you." says the sharks

They then escort her back home; they even stay there as it is way too late and dark for them to go back home. The rest of the evening is peaceful.

Fish sitting

Marlin has to go out today but doesn't want to leave Nemo at home alone with how young he is.

"Daaaaad, I don't want to go," says Nemo

"Well Nemo, I can't leave you home alone; it isn't safe," says Marlin

"I can babysit if he doesn't want to go," says Dory

"Really, Dory? Are you sure?" asks Marlin

"That would be so cool! Please, Dad, please. I will be good, I promise." says Nemo

"...Alright, but Dory is in charge what she says goes," says Marlin

"Sweet. Thanks, dad," says Nemo, hugging him. Marlin smiles and hugs back

"I will be back by dinner," says Marlin

"Alright." They say

Off Marlin goes, Nemo swims about happily.

"Woah, someones excited," says Dory

"Yeah! I love spending time with dad, but his outings are more chores, so it's really boring. I am glad I get to stay home with you, Dory." says Nemo

"Aw. Me too, Nemo." says Dory, "So let's play a game."

"Okay!" says Nemo

"How about you! Hide and go seek! You go hide, and I count, and then after I find you, I will hide, and you find me. It will be so much fun!" says Dory

"Alright! Close your eyes and count to ten!" says Nemo

Nemo swims off but not too far and waits for Dory to start counting and covering her eyes before he hides. She counts to ten and looks about, totally forgetting what she was doing.

"N-Nemo? Oh no, I lost him already! Nemo!" says Dory.

She starts looking for him everywhere, hoping he isn't too far away. She finds him hiding behind some coral.

"Oh, thank god you are okay," says Dory

"Yeah, I am fine. We're playing hide and go seek to remember?" asks Nemo

"Oh, right! Duh forgot," says Dory

"How about we play something else?" asks Nemo

"Okay, what do you want to play?" asks Dory

"How about tag?" asks Nemo

"Ooo sounds like fun!" says Dory

"Great because you're it!" says Nemo

He tags her and swims off. She laughs and goes after him, then tags him.

"I think you're more confused than I am, Nemo, because you're it! Try to catch me!" says Dory

She swims but keeps a slower pace knowing that Nemo is younger than Marlin and should be given a chance. He laughs, giving her chase, it takes him longer, but he does catch her. They play a few rounds until lunchtime than Nemo has a race with her. She loves bonding with him and lets him win.

"I won!" says Nemo

"I see that you did awesomely!" says Dory

"Hey did you let me win?" asks Nemo

"Maybe a little, but that's okay. Maybe one day you will beat me for real," says Dory

"Yeah, and I will get faster and faster!" says Nemo

"That's the spirit. Hungry? I can get us both food." says Dory

"Yeah!" says Nemo

"Great, you wait at home, and I will be right back. I am not going too far. I am a babysitter, so I don't think I should leave you long." says Dory

"Okay, Dory," says Nemo

She smiles and swims off to do so; she comes back after a few minutes with something to eat. They eat up and start playing "red light green light," taking turns being the caller fish. They even have another race where Nemo talks Dory into not letting him win. He doesn't mind losing; he just wants to have some fun with Dory; he really adores her. Soon he gets really tired, and Dory helps him get home for a nap before dinner.

"Today was so much fun," says Nemo with a yawn

"Yeah, it was," says Dory

"Thank you for today, Dory," says Nemo

"Not a problem Nemo, why not take a nap? Your dad will be home soon," says Dory

"Okay," says Nemo

It isn't long before he is out for a nap; Dory smiles and relaxes for a few minutes before Marlin comes home.

"I'm home! Hey Dory, where is Nemo?" asks Marlin

"Welcome home. Oh, he was tuckered out from playing all day, so I helped him to bed for a nap before dinner," says Dory

"He wasn't any trouble, was he?" asks Marlin

"Nah. He was really good; we had a lot of fun. Oh, how was your day?" asks Dory

"It was alright, kind of boring, but I helped who I needed to and got everything done. I am glad everything went well; maybe you can do it again someday," says Marlin

"I would love to!" says Dory

"Great," says Marlin

Soon Nemo wakes up and is happy to tell his dad over dinner his adventures with Dory.

"It sounds like you had a great day," says Marlin

"I did it! Can Dory babysit all the time?" asks Nemo

"I am sure that would be fine," says Marlin

"Yay," says Nemo

They smile and enjoy dinner together.

Overheard Teasing

It was time for a lunch break, and Dory was with Mr. Ray because Mr. Ray wanted to talk to her for a bit; she wasn't in trouble, but he wanted to teach the class without her repeating what he said. In the meantime Pearl, Tad, and Sheldon race Nemo and manage to get far away. However, what they don't know is Nemo learned to swim faster and catches up, but he stays back, hearing them giggle and talk about him.

"I can't believe he is so slow," says Pearl

"He does have that tiny baby fin," says Sheldon

"Yeah, well, I have a tiny tentacle, and I am still faster than him," says Pearl

"I don't have a problem with that. I am more focused on his babysitter," says Tad

"I know, right? Is the four?!" asks Sheldon, sarcastically

They laugh at that; Nemo frowns. He knows they are just teasing, but it is really getting to him.

"Such a baby. Its a wonder his daddy doesn't let him leave without his baba and binky," says Tad

They laugh more, mocking him a little bit. Nemo shakes his head clear and calls out to them. They shut up quickly and smile at him.

"Hey Nemo," they say

They are surprised that he isn't out of breath like normally.

"Your getting better at swimming fast, huh?" asks Sheldon

"Yeah, I have been practicing with Dory. I almost caught up with her," says Nemo

"Y-you did?" asks Pearl

"Yeah," says Nemo, proudly

"Wow." they all say

They get worried that he heard them.

"Um...did you hear anything?" asks Tad

"Hear what?" asks Nemo, playing dumb

"Uh, nothing!" they say

"We better get going; Mr. Ray will be looking for us," says Nemo

So they start back to where the other kids were, and the rest of the day flew by, but the words Tad, Sheldon, and Pearl said stook to Nemo the rest of the day. He went home with Dory that day as Marlin had other things to do, but he does meet up with them for dinner.

"Hey Dory, next few days can you stay home?" asks Nemo

"Uh, sure. But why?" asks Dory, confused

"I just don't want you to go to school with me anymore!" says Nemo

He doesn't want them to worry, so he swims off to bed.

"Nemo!" calls Marlin

He doesn't answer; Marlin and Dory look that way, worried.

"Im sorry, Dory, I don't know where that came from," says Marlin

"Its okay, um...you might have to remind me next few days, but if he doesn't want me there, I won't go," says Dory

She doesn't want to hurt Nemo and can tell from his tone that he is hurting. So the rest of the week and three days into the next one, Dory stays away after being reminded by both Marlin and Nemo that she should stay home for a while. Nemo misses Dory at school, and so don't the other kids, including Pearl, Tad, and Sheldon.

"Hey Nemo, do you know why Dory hasn't been coming to school anymore?" asks Pearl

"I asked her not to anymore," says Nemo

"But why?" asks Sheldon

"Because I am not a baby and don't need a babysitter," says Nemo, finishing his lunch

The three look at each other at that.

"...You heard us the other day, didn't you?" asks Tad

"...Yeah, I did, and I will admit it hurt, but your right. Dory was basically a babysitter, and I don't need that," says Nemo

Thet took a little aback at that; they didn't mean to hurt him or for Dory to disappear.

"Lunch is about over; we better go," says Nemo

"Nemo waits; we're so sorry. We shouldn't have said that" they say at once

"Huh?" asks Nemo

"We were wrong, your not a baby, and Dory is not your babysitter," says Tad

"We were over the top; now we realize that we miss Dory," says Pearl

"Yeah," says the boys

"Please can you get Dory back? We are so sorry, we won't say anything mean like that again," says Sheldon

"Please Nemo, Please," says Pearl and Tad

They beg for a bit; Nemo is confused but thinks about it for a bit.

"Okay, I will ask Dory later. I do feel bad about asking her to stay away," says Nemo

The three grinned at that, and it is good that Nemo thought quickly because Mr. Ray was calling for them.

"Race ya," says Nemo, and off he goes

The other three were stunned for a minute but then laugh and catch up with Nemo. Mr. Ray was happy to see Nemo in a better mood; he looked rather gloomy the past few days. All the kids did, but that is because they missed Dory, but Nemo looked the saddest, like something else was bothering him.

"Nemo," calls Mr. Ray

Nemo swam over to where Mr. Ray was.

"Yeah?" asks Nemo

"Is everything okay?" asks Mr. Ray

"Better than okay," says Nemo. "Oh! Dory may be back tomorrow."

"That's good to hear," says Mr. Ray, "Come on, I think your friends are waiting."

Nemo nods and caught up with his friends, and the rest of the day went smoothly. Later on, Marlin took Nemo home, and Nemo hugs Dory as soon as he gets home.

"Woah hi to you too," says Dory

"I am so sorry for asking to stay away from will you please come back to school," says Nemo

"Uh, sure. Hey! How about tomorrow!" says Dory, excited

"Yay!" says Nemo

"What do we say, Nemo," says Marlin, smiling

"Oh yeah! Thank you, Dory," says Nemo

"Aw, it's not a problem, Nemo," says Dory

He smiles at that, the rest of the evening is peaceful, and the next day everything goes back to normal.

Sleepy Time

It has been a day since they started to live together as close-by neighbors, as Nemo's and Marlin's house would shock her. Dory wakes up early in the morning with Marlin and Nemo, then goes to school with Nemo. It is odd that she wants to go to elementary school as an elementary student, but Mr. Ray and Marlin let her do it, not sure how to tell her that this is more for children who don't know what anything really is. Then Dory goes back home to try to help Marlin out at home, when Mr. Ray has something to do that is too far and knows that Dory will get lost, especially with Nemo needing special attention. As Nemo missed a few days of school, Mr. Ray has been trying to get him to catch up, and that is hard to do when you are teaching twenty students and helping another student on top of helping an adult getting distracted on every little thing.

"Dory? Aren't you suppose to be at school right now?" asks Marlin

"Mr. Ray said that he has a special assignment for me today," says Dory

"What's that?" asks Marlin, afraid to know the answer

He knows Mr. Ray wouldn't turn her away and hurt her feelings, but who knows what she got herself into today.

"I am to help you today! While he helps Nemo!" says Dory

"That's a great idea!" says Marlin, sighing with relief

"Yup! So what do I have to do today?" asks Dory

"Well, uh. I was actually going to clean up some debris from around the path, Nemo likes playing outside, and I know that there are rough edges. I don't want him to get hurt on anything, you see?" says Marlin

"Oh! I can do that, just tell me where everything goes, and I will take care of it!" says Dory

"Really?" asks Marlin

"Yeah!" says Dory

"Well. I do need to run some errands in town today..okay Dory. Listen, if you see anything colorful and smooth, it goes in the good pile here next to the house. If you see anything rough and full of edges, toss it in the coral for now, and I will take care of it when I get back." says Marlin

"I can handle that!" says Dory

"Great! I will be back in two hours," says Marlin

He left, hoping he was making the right decision instead of sending her off into town. He shook his head, knowing that would be worse.

"Okay, colorful and smooth near the house, rough edges in the coral," says Dory

She starts saying that to herself as she works, and then the commands get mixed up; while she works, everything gets sorted backward when Marlin comes back and notices that the piles are mixed together.

"Uh. Dory...what happened?" asks Marlin

"I'm sorry.. so sorry... I forgot what you said, and it turned into this. I am so sorry. I tried to fix it, and it got worse." says Dory, very apologetic

Marlin sighs figured that would happen, and soothe her.

"It's alright, let me put things up, and I will help you, okay?" asks Marlin

"Alright," says Dory

They get to work getting things done and ready for Nemo after they get him and go back home. After that, they would play until exhaustion, eat dinner, and go to bed. This sort of pattern would go on for a while. Nemo and Dory would get up and go to school; then, Dory would be sent home to do some sort of task for Marlin. Marlin and Mr. Ray liked this pattern, so didn't Nemo because that meant he got to bond with Dory more and more. It went on like that for four days, then one night, Dory's body got tired of not swimming everywhere without going anywhere, so it woke her up without waking her and made her move and start swimming. There was a ruckus that woke up Marlin and Dory as they slept, and they noticed that Dory was gone.

"Dory?!" they called

They looked about looking for any sign of her, and Nemo finally spotted her.

"Dad! There!" says Nemo, pointing her out

They swim over to her calling her name, but every time they did, she wouldn't answer them.

"Dory?" asks Nemo when they reach her

"Her eyes are closed, Nemo. I think she is sleep swimming," says Marlin

"What is sleep swimming?" asks Nemo

"Sleep swimming is where your body wakes up on its' own and moves you without knowing," says Marlin

"Then why not wake her and have her swim home?" asks Nemo

"Because that is dangerous, just have to guide her home," says Marlin

So they gently turn her around and start her the way home.

"Why is she sleep swimming?" asks Nemo

"She isn't used to staying home in one place, Nemo. So her body is telling her to keep swimming for some reason. She didn't have a home before this one. She would swim from one place to the next." says Marlin

"Will she ever not do this?" asks Nemo

"I don't know, son. We just have to wake up and guide her home," says Marlin

"What if...we wake up too late and she is too far gone?" asks Nemo, worried

Marlin looked at Nemo as he tucks Dory back into bed. He pats his head and helps Nemo back into their bed.

"I won't let that happen, I promise," says Marlin

"*smiles* Alright, Dad. *yawn* Good night," says Nemo

"*Smile* Good night, Nemo," says Marlin

The two fell asleep; for the next week, Marlin and Nemo would continue putting Dory back to bed some nights, stopping her before she got two minutes from her house. Finally, her body stopped sleepwalking, and she stayed put, but they checked on her for a week just to be sure. Marlin managed to keep his promise to Nemo; Nemo snuggles Marlin.

"What's this for, hmm?" asks Marlin

"For keeping your promise and Dory with us. I knew you could do it. I love you." says Nemo

Marlin smiles and snuggles Nemo back, holding him close.

"I love you too," says Marlin